Family work in mental health
A skills approach

For the full range of M&K Publishing books please visit our website:
www.mkupdate.co.uk

Family work in mental health
A skills approach

Edited by
Nicola Evans

Family work in mental health:
A skills approach
Nicola Evans
ISBN: 978-1-905539-65-9
First published 2019

All rights reserved. No part of this publication may be reproduced, stored in a retrieval system, or transmitted in any form or by any means, electronic, mechanical, photocopying, recording or otherwise, without either the prior permission of the publishers or a licence permitting restricted copying in the United Kingdom issued by the Copyright Licensing Agency, 90 Tottenham Court Road, London, W1T 4LP. Permissions may be sought directly from M&K Publishing, phone: 01768 773030, fax: 01768 781099 or email: publishing@mkupdate.co.uk

Any person who does any unauthorised act in relation to this publication may be liable to criminal prosecution and civil claims for damages.

British Library Cataloguing in Publication Data
A catalogue record for this book is available from the British Library

Notice
Clinical practice and medical knowledge constantly evolve. Standard safety precautions must be followed, but, as knowledge is broadened by research, changes in practice, treatment and drug therapy may become necessary or appropriate. Readers must check the most current product information provided by the manufacturer of each drug to be administered and verify the dosages and correct administration, as well as contraindications. It is the responsibility of the practitioner, utilising the experience and knowledge of the patient, to determine dosages and the best treatment for each individual patient. Any brands mentioned in this book are as examples only and are not endorsed by the publisher. Neither the publisher nor the authors assume any liability for any injury and/or damage to persons or property arising from this publication.

To contact M&K Publishing write to:
M&K Update Ltd · The Old Bakery · St. John's Street
Keswick · Cumbria CA12 5AS
Tel: 01768 773030 · Fax: 01768 781099
publishing@mkupdate.co.uk
www.mkupdate.co.uk

Designed and typeset by Mary Blood
Printed in Scotland by Bell & Bain

Contents

Contributors: *vii*

Introduction: *ix*
An introduction to family work in mental health
Nicola Evans

Chapter 1: *1*
The application of family-centred care in the field of mental health nursing
Jane Davies and Ben Hannigan

Chapter 2: *15*
Understanding and assessing the needs of families and carers
John Hyde

Chapter 3: *31*
Working with families affected by psychosis
Alicia Stringfellow

Chapter 4: *39*
Parents with mental health issues – thinking about the whole family
Nicola Evans

Chapter 5: *51*
Understanding moment-by-moment interactions in families: assessment and treatment utilising a domains framework
S. Riley, J. Hill, H. Lee and P. Tranter

Chapter 6: *67*
Perinatal mental health and working with families
Sue Barker

Chapter 7: *83*
Family support and involvement in secure mental health services
Mick McKeown, Fiona Jones, Sue Stewart and Sheena Foster

Chapter 8: 103
Substance misuse, alcohol and working with families
Gemma Stacey-Emile

Chapter 9: 115
Working with military veterans
Clare Crole-Rees, Neil Kitchiner and Dean Whybrow

Chapter 10: 127
Working with families affected by dementia
Mandy King

Index: 144

Contributors

Dr Sue Barker was a mental health lecturer at Cardiff University and is now enjoying retirement.

Clare Crole-Rees is a registered counselling psychologist and works in the School of Psychology, Cardiff University.

Dr Jane Davies is Senior lecturer and RCBC Postdoctoral Fellow in children and young people's nursing at Cardiff University.

Dr Nicola Evans is a Reader at Cardiff University, specialising in children's mental health.

Sheena Foster is a carer and works with the RCPsych in the Quality Network.

Professor Ben Hannigan is a mental health nurse, researcher and teacher and is currently Professor of Mental Health Nursing at Cardiff University.

Professor Jonathan Hill is Professor of Child and Adolescent Psychiatry at Reading University.

John Hyde is a mental health nurse and lecturer at Cardiff University.

Fiona Jones has lived experience of secure care and working as a researcher.

Amanda King is a mental health nurse and lecturer in Cardiff University.

Dr Neil Kitchiner is a Principal Clinician & Honorary Research Fellow in Cardiff and Vale University Health Board Veterans Service.

Heather Lee is a Highly Specialised Family and Systemic Psychotherapist MSC, BN (hons) BSC (hons). Currently she works in North East Wales CAMHS services as lead for family therapy.

Professor Mick McKeown is a mental health nurse, educator and researcher at University of Central Lancashire.

Steve Riley is a Consultant Nurse and Systemic/Family Psychotherapist, having worked within specialist CAMHS in Betsi Cadwalladar University Health Board.

Gemma Stacey-Emile is a Lecturer in mental health nursing at Cardiff University.

Sue Stewart is a parent carer whose journey has been from a Mental Health Carer to a Forensic Carer.

Alicia Stringfellow is a Lecturer in mental health nursing at Cardiff University.

Paul Tranter is a Consultant Family & Systemic Psychotherapist working in Betsi Cadwalladar University Health Board.

Dean Whybrow is a Lecturer in mental health nursing at Cardiff University.

An introduction to family work in mental health

Nicola Evans

Throughout my mental health career, I have been interested in working with families. In many specialities within mental health, this is an area of work that practitioners appear to shy away from, perhaps because they lack the knowledge or skill to incorporate this important aspect into their clinical work. Maybe, within some health professions, we are encouraged to think about the person seeking help as our first priority; the context in which they live then becomes a secondary consideration.

However, there is now good evidence that working with families can be helpful to the person experiencing the mental health issue. For example, we know that offering family intervention for people with psychosis can in some cases reduce the relapse rate. We also know that working with the whole family can be helpful in reducing the stress or burden on carers – for example, in families of people with dementia. We are also aware that families themselves seek help, support and information and warrant services in their own right. In some countries, this has led to legislation acknowledging the rights of families to have their own needs assessed and met through the introduction of the Carers Act 2014 (England) and the Carers Strategies (Wales) Measure 2010, which clearly state that health professionals need to attend to the needs of family and carers.

Carers and families also tell us they want to be more involved where possible. There are specific organisations to inform and support carers such as Rethink Mental Illness (a UK-based mental health charity that has specific resources for carers) and the National Network of Carers Associations, Australia (which includes carers of people with mental illness).

So, we know there is evidence that working with families of people with mental issues is helpful and we know families want to be involved, but unless healthcare practitioners have specific knowledge and training in working with families, it appears that this approach is not routinely offered. Sveinbjarnardottir *et al.* (2011) found that when a sample of mental health nurses were trained in a model of family systems nursing, based on the Calgary Family Assessment and Family Intervention models (Wright &Leahey 2009), they saw the families as less 'burdensome'. This change in attitude enabled nurses to think of families in a more positive light and created a more optimistic outlook for therapeutic working with families in this study.

Given the need for family work in mental health, and the reluctance of many mental health professionals to engage in that work due to lack of confidence, knowledge and skills, this book aims to discuss approaches to working with families of people with mental health issues in a number of contexts. The contributors have tried to bring together a range of ways in which mental health practitioners can work with children, adults and families who access mental health services. As with all novel clinical approaches, it is important that such interventions are discussed with the families themselves at the outset, involving them as equal partners in a collaborative relationship. When care is organised by a multidisciplinary team, any proposed family work should be discussed within the wider care context. This should help ensure its relevance, prevent duplication and lead to the provision of seamless care. Effective clinical supervision will help promote a good-quality clinical service by enabling the practitioner to engage in reflective practice and seek guidance when necessary.

Where possible, illustrative examples have been used to illustrate how family work can be implemented, showing the application of a particular theory or model in a hypothetical case.

Families: Structure, roles, construction

When we think about families, each of us may have a different idea of what the term 'family' means. Its meaning is changing over time, and can differ according to a person's culture, religion and personal philosophy. When talking to people with mental health issues about their family, it may therefore be helpful to start by asking who they consider to be part of their immediate and wider family, and how they are connected. For instance, a family might mean a group of individuals living under one roof, demonstrating reciprocal affections and loyalties (Carter & McGoldrick 2005). Such a group may have a sense of belonging with one another, and perhaps an agreed system of managing finances and allocating chores, with a shared history, family rituals and philosophy on life (Fawcett 1993). In the 21st century there are many different types of family units and the traditional nuclear family model is less common these days. It is now customary to have families consisting of half-siblings, step-relations, adopted or fostered children, and adults cohabiting without being married. The boundary of the family unit is less easily defined, with partners not necessarily living in the same household or with individuals sharing their time between households. Rather than worrying about how to 'draw the boundary line' around the family, it may be more natural for the healthcare practitioner to ask the person accessing mental health services who they would consider to be in the family. The practitioner could perhaps construct a genogram with them, and thus create an opportunity to think about the family, its construction, how people interact with one another and the important relationships within that family.

We hope this book will inspire you to consider working more with families, think about the individual in front of you in the context of their family relationships, and explore ways of working with the wider family unit. We have drawn on interventions or approaches where there is an established evidence base – as in Chapter 3, where we look at interventions for families with a member who experiences psychosis. There are also new approaches (such as the domains framework, described in Chapter 6) which invite us to think differently about the communication between parent and child. Although problem-solving strategies are commonly used in mental health, we present two different approaches to therapeutic problem-solving with families in Chapters 3 and 10, showing the value of adapting such collaborative approaches to meet the particular needs of individual families.

References

Carter, B. & McGoldrick, M. (eds) (2005). *The Expanded Family Life Cycle: Individual, Family and Social Perspectives*. Boston: Allyn & Bacon.

Fawcett, C.S. (1993). *Family Psychiatric Nursing*. St Louis: Mosby.

Sveinbjarnardottir, E.K., Svavarsdottir, E.K. & Saveman, B.I. (2011). Nurses' attitudes towards the importance of families in psychiatric care following an educational and training intervention program. *Journal of Psychiatric and Mental Health Nursing*. **18**, 895–903.

Wright, L.M. & Leahey, J.M. (2009). *Nurses and Families: A Guide to Family Assessment and Intervention*. 5th edn. Philadelphia: FA Davis Company.

Chapter 1
The application of family-centred care in the field of mental health nursing

Jane Davies and Ben Hannigan

Introduction

This chapter begins with an outline of the philosophy of family-centred care (FCC) as it has evolved within the children's and young people's nursing field. We then discuss the current position of this popular approach in relation to mental health nursing as a whole. A relatively short history of, and context for, this way of providing and managing care will set the scene for the rest of the chapter.

Whilst the literature argues that family-centred approaches offer some benefits, there is also evidence of various challenges. If not identified and managed effectively, these can significantly affect the individual and family experience. The most frequently cited benefits and challenges in the evidence base will be briefly discussed, after which an alternative approach to family-centred care will be discussed.

This will be followed by an attempt to frame a family-centred model of care within child and adolescent mental health services (CAMHS), and in the context of mental health services for adults. The aim will be to consider how using a family-centred care model could help to enhance provision for people of all ages needing mental healthcare and treatment. It is envisaged that this will contribute to future thinking about the possible usefulness of transferring a well-established model found within the children's physical healthcare field into the area of mental health nursing.

Aims and learning outcomes

This chapter aims to offer an overview of the family-centred care model that is commonly found in children's services and consider its application to mental healthcare. Having read the chapter, the reader will have:

- An understanding of family-centred care
- Ideas as to how this approach might be applied in mental health.

Family-centred care

The philosophy of family-centred care has not had a particularly long history in children's and young people's nursing. In the 1950s, for example, children would often be taken to hospital for an elective procedure, where they would be left (usually by their mother) until they were ready to be discharged. Only a limited amount of time was permitted for visiting during this period. It was not until the early 1950s that approaches to the care of children slowly began to change. In his publication *Child Care and the Growth of Love*, John Bowlby asserted a number of principles relating to the importance of children being supported by their families. Most importantly perhaps, he referred to the adverse effects of separating a child from their mother, resulting in what is commonly referred to today as 'separation anxiety' (Bowlby 1953). This proved to be a catalyst for later work, including that of Robertson and Robertson (1971), which focused on the care of young children in hospital. Despite not agreeing with some of Bowlby's work they acknowledged, 'we continue to share his concern about the potential harm associated with early separation from the mother' (p. 313).

Additionally, a timely policy document from the Ministry of Health, published in 1959, known commonly in children and young people's nursing literature as the Platt report, studied the welfare of sick children in hospital in terms of the specific arrangements that were made for them. These considerations were distinct from the medical and nursing treatment they received. The Platt report also published recommendations which were communicated to hospital authorities at the time. In recent years (particularly from the mid-1980s onwards), there has been a recognition that caring for children and young people requires not just being concerned with 'managing' the child or young person in terms of their presenting symptoms, rather there has been a concerted move towards family involvement in care. It is now well recognised that the context in which the everyday lives of children and young people takes place is usually dependent to some extent on parents, carers and sometimes the wider family.

The context of family-centred care

When a child or young person is unwell, families (not unreasonably) usually experience a degree of stress. Parents or carers are likely to be concerned and anxious about the cause of the illness and will be keen to know what the future holds. Families will commonly have a number of commitments and these will often include caring for other children or older people in the family. Financial and work commitments may also be a worry, thus increasing stress levels (Tallon *et al.* 2015). A young person's illness will cause family members to lose sleep, causing tiredness.

It is also sometimes the case that families find themselves in an unfamiliar environment, which makes them feel unsure, confused and lacking the power, knowledge and influence to manage their lives. In contrast, the professionals caring for the families are in familiar surroundings and have expert knowledge of the events which are taking place. This situation can lead to professionals to 'taking over' and potentially excluding families from decisions about care – not always intentionally. It is against this backdrop that we should consider how best children and young people might be cared for, whilst recognising the importance of family involvement and how this can help in the care process. The key factors in family-centred care are highlighted in Table 1.1. below.

Table 1.1: Elements of family-centred care

The following elements were proposed by the Institute for Family-centred Care and cited in Shields (2010):
● Recognising the family as a constant in the child's life
● Facilitating parent–professional collaboration at all levels of healthcare
● Honouring the racial, ethnic, cultural, and socio-economic diversity of families
● Recognising family strengths and individuality and respecting different methods of coping
● Sharing complete and unbiased information with families on a continuous basis
● Encouraging and facilitating family-to-family support and networking
● Responding to child and family developmental needs as part of healthcare practices
● Adopting policies and practices that provide families with emotional and financial support
● Designing healthcare that is flexible, culturally competent, and responsive to family needs.

Benefits of family-centred care

Over the last three decades, the concept of family-centred care has been acknowledged as a key feature of healthcare practice in children's and young people's nursing. Many practitioners have espoused the benefits of family-centred care in planning, implementing and evaluating care for children and young people. Despite this, no empirical evidence has been provided that family-centred care makes a difference to clinical outcomes for children, young people and families (Shields *et al.* 2007, Shields *et al.* 2012).

Nevertheless, Coyne (2013) acknowledges that family-centred care is thought to be beneficial for a number of other reasons, including the positive effects of bonding between the child and family, and the reduction of the negative effects of hospitalisation (such as the reduction of anxiety) and an increase in satisfaction regarding the care received. Similarly, in a systematic review undertaken by Power and Franck (2008), it was demonstrated that parents felt they benefited from making a contribution to family-centred care and this positivity also affected the child and the healthcare professionals. Another view offered by Smith *et al.* (2002) presented the concept of family-centred care as a continuum, where care could be nurse-led and then move to an equal balance between the nurse and the family, ultimately resulting in family-led care. The benefit of such a continuum is that families and healthcare professionals can move from one position to another, based on the changing needs of the child and family.

Challenges to family-centred care

Undeniably there have been challenges to the concept of family-centred care. This is partly because significant changes have been implemented over a relatively short period of time. The whole philosophy of care changed from one of not involving families towards a very clear expectation that family involvement would be central to the care of children and young people. Callery and Smith (1991) were particularly interested in how roles between parents and professionals were negotiated in order to achieve a family-centred approach. In a small study they identified a number of factors that could potentially create barriers to a family-centred approach. For example, they referred to the unequal power balance between parents and professionals sometimes rendering negotiation difficult, with parents often being placed in a weaker position when deciding how care should be best organised.

Brown and Ritchie (1990) also reported that the attitude of nurses could significantly affect the power balance in the nurse/family relationship. They comment that parents are judged in terms of their values and this in turn makes a difference to the way in which healthcare professionals behave towards parents. This judgement could manifest itself in a number of ways, which might include negative attitudes towards different religions, cultural practice, family structure and background. Furthermore, Callery and Smith (1991) suggest that several other barriers exist, due to the child becoming unwell. These include the stress created as a result of the illness, the anxiety relating to the potential outcome of the illness, the uncertainty surrounding the diagnosis of illness, and the fatigue sometimes created by looking after a sick child at home prior to admission to hospital (Callery & Smith 1991).

Similarly, Knafl *et al.* (1992) explored parents' views, which led to suggestions about how to establish a positive working relationship between healthcare professionals and families. These suggestions included, for instance, providing mutually useful communication between healthcare professionals and parents, ensuring that information is exchanged effectively, helping parents to achieve competence where relevant in aspects of care-giving, and establishing a relationship with the child who is being cared for. Chapados et al. (2009) also found that families sometimes felt overwhelmed by their care-giving responsibilities and were afraid of making mistakes due to a lack of competence.

Furthermore, Shields (2010) questioned the usefulness of family-centred care. This author reported evidence of parents being left to care for their child with little help from staff, commenting that parents felt they were being judged for their level of involvement, particularly in cases where they were unable to stay with their child. In conclusion, Shields (2010) suggested a new, more effective model of care. More recently, it has been acknowledged by Tallon et al. (2015) that doubts still exist as to the effectiveness of family-centred care, in view of the fact that there is still no empirical evidence that children and young people achieve better clinical outcomes as a result of this approach.

Nevertheless Tallon et al. (2015) do not call for an abandonment of the concept; rather, they suggest an alternative model. This model takes into account a variety of disciplines which they claim can change the practice of nursing in this context. Tallon and colleagues examined literature from fields including psychology, anthropology, sociology and neuroscience. Their key argument is that family-centred care for children and young people with serious illness and long-term conditions needs to accommodate many factors, in addition to the theory of attachment (which is considered to be central). These additional factors include the 'benefits of applying a bioecological model of human development, the family and community resource framework, allostatic load and biological embedding, empowerment and the nurse family partnership' (p. 1432).

The bioecological model of human development, first proposed by Bronfenbrenner and Ceci (1994), highlights the biological, social and psychological processes that influence development. These include perspectives on micro, meso and macro systems, how development is influenced by environmental contexts and how these systems and contexts change over time. Tallon et al. (2015) argue that there is evidence supporting the use of this model because social health can be very dependent on these structural factors. They emphasise the importance of the family and community resource framework and the relevance of a number of family issues when caring for a seriously ill child. These include factors like the knowledge of the parents, the well-being of mothers, financial constraints, access to support and the centrality of human and social capital.

Individuals can develop biological mechanisms to cope with stress. However, in situations where stress is experienced over a long period of time, this can have negative consequences for the individual (McEwan & Seeman 1999). This can of course affect children and young people as well as parents. Finally, the concept of nurse–family partnerships is highlighted. These relationships between nurses and families play a vital part in providing effective care. When such partnerships are developed with a focus on equality, listening and valuing what parents say, it is more likely that individual health needs will be met. This is extremely important in children's nursing where there can be high levels of vulnerability and dependence can be high.

In order to build a positive therapeutic relationship, it is essential to take the time to find out about how individual families are structured, and what their socioeconomic and psychosocial characteristics are. The future of effective family-centred care perhaps rests on a combination of its original premise and approaches, coupled with further thinking as identified by Tallon *et al.* (2015). In the context of this chapter, our thoughts now turn to how we might usefully think about family-centred care in the field of mental health nursing across the lifespan. To help us think about how this model might work, the checklist in Table 1.2 below might offer a useful starting point.

Table 1.2: An alternative way to think about family-centred care *(Tallon et al. 2015)*

These are additional factors in providing effective family-centred care:
● Application of respectful, reflective active listening with a view to completing an effective assessment
● Attention to the developmental needs of each individual
● Prompt assessment to consider the biological, psychological, psychosocial, demographic and socioeconomic issues which are central to each individual child or young person and their family
● Acknowledgement and measurement of the stress (allostatic load) in both children and young people and their families
● Development of a plan which contains a continuum of care, ranging from nurse-led activity to family-led activity, with a view to providing flexibility and movement along the continuum of care as well as an agreed balance of power
● Continuous evaluation of care to meet the changing needs of each individual and family.

Family-centred mental healthcare for children and young people

It is estimated that 1 in 10 children and young people between the ages of 5 and 16 in the UK experiences a mental health difficulty (Green *et al.* 2005). Most are supported by their families and by practitioners who do not specialise in mental healthcare, typically working in primary care settings, schools, and youth and social services agencies. This is often referred to as 'tier 1' within the UK, using the tiered approach commonly found in children and young people's mental health services (CAMHS) and summarised in Table 1.3 below:

Table 1.3: The tiered approach in CAMHS
(Wales Audit Office/Healthcare Inspectorate Wales 2009)

Tier 1: Services provided by professionals whose main role and training is not in mental health. These may include GPs, health visitors, paediatricians, social workers, teachers, youth workers and juvenile justice workers.
Tier 2: Services provided by specialist trained mental health professionals, working primarily on their own. Tier 2 also consists of those practitioners and services from specialist CAMHS that provide initial contacts and assessments of children and young people and their families.
Tier 3: More specialised services provided by multidisciplinary teams (MDTs), according to the complexity and severity of need.
Tier 4: Very specialised services in residential, day-patient or outpatient settings for children and adolescents with severe and/or complex problems.

Within specialist child and adolescent mental health services around the world (tier 2 and above, using UK terminology), the phrase 'family centred care' is sometimes used alongside other terms with similar or overlapping meanings such as 'family focused' and (in North America particularly) 'wraparound' and 'systems of care' (MacKean *et al.* 2012). The language used is important, and care needs to be taken when identifying innovations representing genuine developments in family-centred centre (as explained at the beginning of this chapter). Terms like 'family engagement' are sometimes used to refer to efforts to simply encourage families to attend appointments and follow professionally prescribed plans of treatment (e.g. Gopalan *et al.* 2010), rather than attempts to create services which are more profoundly family- and child-centred.

In MacKean and colleagues' (2012) formulation, a shift towards a family-centred approach in child and adolescent mental health services implies reorientations in ways of working at every level, representing a major departure from traditional models of organising and providing care. This ranges from the national level at the very top, right down to face-to-face individual care at the bottom. These changes are needed in order to forge more collaborative relationships with families and young people throughout the care system. As MacKean *et al.* (2012) observe, this demands attention to national policies, local organisational procedures and to everyday professional practice and values.

Globally, Canada (where MacKean and colleagues are based) stands out as a country in which particularly interesting reorientations of this type are taking place. In a review compiled by the Ontario Centre of Excellence for Child and Youth Mental Health (2017), evidence was brought together relating to developments in 'family engagement' as an approach located within a broader family-centred philosophy of care. In this context, family-centred care means much more than simply encouraging appointment attendance and treatment sign-up, as it is interpreted by Gopalan *et al.* (2010). Instead, it embraces active collaboration and participation, requiring support by leaders, sufficient resources, community involvement, the recognition of family (as well as professional) expertise, inclusivity and the sharing of power (Ontario Centre of Excellence for Child and Youth Mental Health 2017). This review concludes that evidence now exists that family engagement approaches bring benefits not only to young people and their families but also to whole systems. Elsewhere in Canada, sustained partnerships have developed between service providers and universities to organise, provide and evaluate family- and child-centred approaches (McCay *et al.* 2015).

For small numbers of young people, as Table 1.3 above shows, care is provided in inpatient or other residential services. At tier 4, family-centred care may face challenges due to geographical distance, making it difficult for families to keep in touch with young people who may be far from their homes (Hannigan *et al.* 2015). However, hospital-based examples from around the world can be found of family-centred care in action. For instance, Regan *et al.* (2006) describe a detailed case study on introducing and evaluating family-centred care in a child assessment unit in Cambridge Hospital, Massachusetts. At the time of publication, this was a service for under-12s with trauma-related, anxiety, mood and other mental health difficulties. Stays for young people could be as long as nine months. Family-centred care was introduced as part of a wider organisational and cultural change, involving a move away from the control and containment of young people in favour of 'nurturance, opportunities to learn and teach, and providing choices based on individual needs' (p. 35).

Three key components of a family centred approach informed this change: a commitment to collaborative problem-solving; having open visiting hours for parents; and the introduction of trauma-informed procedures. Collaborative problem-solving involved attempts to better understand young people's actions and to build relationships, rather than responding to behavioural transgressions in ways that might be interpreted as punitive. The move towards open hours meant lifting restrictions on parental visiting times, with the aim of increasing opportunities for consultation between staff and families and for the fostering of partnerships. Trauma-sensitive protocols developed by Regan *et al.* (2006) recognised that many of the young people in the unit had been exposed to violence, and these protocols were introduced to encourage trust and safety.

In recent years, developments in children and young people's mental health services have included the introduction of intensive community teams providing interprofessional support for young people who might otherwise be in residential or hospital care, and their families. Case studies reveal explicit shifts towards more family-centred approaches to care, with an example being the establishment of a community intensive therapy team (CITT) in south Wales, UK (Darwish *et al.* 2006). Reasons for the establishment of this new team, described as sitting at the interface of tiers 3 and 4, included a desire to avoid hospital admission wherever possible, in recognition of the dislocation this causes as it removes young people from their everyday contacts with family, friends and education. Part of the CITT philosophy is the opportunity that intensive home-based intervention offers for ongoing collaboration with families or other carers, who might otherwise be marginalised if care is provided in institutional settings.

Family-centred mental health care for adults

Across adult mental health services, more attention is being paid to involving (and collaborating with) families in the provision of care, a process which reflects the historic shift in the provision of care from institutions to the community (Hannigan & Allen 2006). In fact, the term 'family-centred care' is rarely used in a direct way in this context, although many of the principles of family-centred care (as summarised earlier in Tables 1.1. and 1.2) will resonate with nurses caring for adults with mental health problems.

Broadly speaking, family involvement with people with severe mental health problems can be thought of as a continuum, beginning with providing general information on service availability and progressing through to specialised clinical care involving psychoeducation and family interventions drawing on psychological theory (Eassom *et al.* 2014). The current NICE guidance draws on evidence that families and carers often feel poorly informed about the mental health care and treatment their loved ones receive, and struggle to keep in touch with services (NICE 2011). In a recent study of care planning and coordination in community mental health settings in England and Wales, carers reported varying degrees of involvement in discussions and decision-making with professionals. They also reported tensions between the dual aims of increasing family involvement while also preserving confidentiality (Simpson *et al.* 2016). In a related study investigating care planning and coordination in inpatient mental health services, carers described high-quality care being provided but also said there were limited opportunities for them to be involved (Simpson *et al.* 2017).

One very well-developed area of clinical research within the mental health field relates to psychosocial family interventions (see Chapter 3). Early observations on the links between family environment and the recurrence of psychotic experiences and subsequent return to hospital were made in the 1960s and 1970s – with criticism, hostility and over-involvement implicated in increasing the risk of relapse (Brown *et al.* 1972). Psychosocial approaches, including behavioural family interventions, have been widely investigated by research teams around the world and are associated with a reduction in rates of relapse and hospital readmission (Pharoah *et al.* 2010). Family interventions of this type are characterised by the creation of close therapeutic alliances, the provision of help to modify home environments by reducing levels of anger and hostility and promoting practical problem-solving. Their use is now endorsed in guidelines published by the National Institute for Health and Care Excellence (NICE 2014). However, there are many barriers to the routine implementation of specialist family interventions, including unsympathetic organisational cultures, lack of access to training and supervision, and limited whole-team commitment (Eassom *et al.* 2014).

The broad principles of collaborating with, and directly involving, families in decisions around mental health care are also strongly endorsed in philosophies, services and standards relating to the care of older adults. For example, Kitwood's ideas about person-centred care for people with dementia (Kitwood 1997), and contemporary approaches to 'personalisation', both include commitments to supporting and involving family carers as well as individuals (Manthorpe & Samsi 2016).

The idea of supporting family carers is also emphasised by the emergence of Admiral nurses, a group supported by Dementia UK and specifically equipped with skills and competency in helping families caring for people with memory-related problems (Dewing & Traynor 2005). Within mental health services for older people more generally, prevailing clinical standards are clear that family carers should receive adequate information and support, and have opportunities to be involved in decisions about care (NICE 2016).

To close this chapter, we present a brief case study, derived from research completed by one of the authors (BH), which exemplifies the application of family-centred approaches to the care of a young adult with severe mental health difficulties. The reader is invited to respond to a series of questions on this case study.

Illustrative case study of family-centred approach with a young adult with severe mental health difficulties

'Lenny' was a young man who participated in a research project investigating the provision of interprofessional care for people with severe mental health problems (Hannigan & Allen 2013). Lenny had a long, fragmented, experience of using mental health services. Members of his care team had historically struggled to meet his complex needs, which included depression and self-harm, substance misuse and – crucially – family conflict. A mental health worker with new responsibilities to coordinate Lenny's care took the initiative to negotiate a new plan of care which, in his words, included the provision of 'insight-oriented' family therapy. This involved work to develop a strong therapeutic alliance between Lenny's care coordinator, Lenny himself and his parents.

The work of family carers was therefore embraced as a central, indispensable, part of Lenny's care and treatment.

Reflection

If you were asked to work with Lenny and his family, how might you involve all members of the family in negotiating a collaborative care plan? What might the mental health worker have meant by 'insight-oriented' therapy? What knowledge and skill would a practitioner need in order to foster and sustain a strong therapeutic alliance with Lenny and his family?

Conclusion

Family-centred care emerged specifically in the context of children and young people's nursing. In this chapter we have shown how some of the core principles underpinning this approach inform, or have kinship with, approaches to working with families in the context of mental health care delivered across the lifespan. Families often play a key role in supporting loved ones who are experiencing distress. When asked, family members will typically say they welcome opportunities to be listened to by practitioners and to be involved in decision-making.

The evidence we have drawn on in this chapter is that professionals often share this wish but struggle (for a whole range of reasons) to translate family-oriented approaches to mental health care into everyday practice. The challenge remains, then, to continue the search for ways of maximising family involvement. Family-centred care, in the context of children and young people's care, offers a set of principles that might usefully be transferred to the care of all people living with mental health difficulties.

References

Bronfenbrenner, U. & Ceci, S.J. (1994). Nature-nurture reconceptualised in developmental perspective: a bioecological model. *Psychological Review.* **101**, 586.

Brown, G.W., Birley, J.L.T. and Wing, J.K. (1972). Influence of family life on the course of schizophrenic disorders: a replication. *British Journal of Psychiatry.* **121** (562), 241–58.

Brown, J. & Ritchie, J. (1990). Nurses' perceptions of parents and nurse roles in caring for hospitalized children. *Children's Healthcare.* **19**, 28–36.

Bowlby, J. (1953). *Child Care and the Growth of Love.* Harmondsworth: Penguin.

Callery, P. & Smith, L. (1991). A study of role negotiation between nurses and the parents of hospitalised children. *Journal of Advanced Nursing.* **16**, 772–81.

Chapados, C., Pineault, R., Tourigny, J. & Vandal, S. (2009). Perceptions of parents' participation in the care of their child undergoing day surgery: Pilot-study. *Issues in Comprehensive Pediatric Nursing.* **25** (1), 59–70.

Coyne, I. (2013). Families and healthcare-professionals' perspectives and expectation of family centred care: hidden expectations and unclear roles. *Health Expectations.* **18**, 796–808.

Darwish, A., Salmon, G., Ahuja, A. & Steed, L. (2006). The community intensive therapy team: development and philosophy of a new service. *Clinical Child Psychology and Psychiatry.* **11** (4), 591–605.

Dewing, J. & Traynor, V. (2005). Admiral nursing competency project: Practice development and action research. *Journal of Clinical Nursing.* **14** (6), 695–703.

Eassom, E., Giacco, D., Dirik, A. & Priebe, S. (2014). Implementing family involvement in the treatment of patients with psychosis: a systematic review of facilitating and hindering factors. *BMJ Open.* **4** (10), e006108.

Gopalan, G., Goldstein, L., Klingenstein, K., Sicher, C., Blake, C. & McKay, M.M. (2010). Engaging families into child mental health treatment: updates and special considerations. *Journal of the Canadian Academy of Child and Adolescent Psychiatry.* **19** (3), 182–96.

Green, H., McGinnity, A., Meltzer, H., Ford, T. & Goodman, R. (2005) *Mental Health of Children and Young People in Great Britain, 2004.* Basingstoke: Palgrave Macmillan.

Hannigan, B. & Allen, D. (2006). Complexity and change in the United Kingdom's system of mental healthcare. *Social Theory & Health.* **4** (3), 244–63.

Hannigan, B. & Allen, D. (2013). Complex caring trajectories in community mental health: contingencies, divisions of labor and care coordination. *Community Mental Health Journal.* **49** (4), 380–88.

Hannigan, B., Edwards, D., Evans, N., Gillen, E., Longo, M., Pryjmachuk, S. & Trainor, G. (2015). An evidence synthesis of risk identification, assessment and management for young people using tier 4 inpatient child and adolescent mental health services. *Health Services and Delivery Research.* **3**, 22.

Kitwood, T. (1997). *Dementia Reconsidered: The Person Comes First.* Buckingham: Open University Press.

Knafl, K., Breitmayer, B., Gallo, A. & Zoeller, L. (1992). Parents' views of healthcare providers: An exploration of the components of a positive working relationship. *Children's Healthcare.* **21** (2), 90–92.

MacKean, G., Spragins, W., L'Heureux, L., Popp, J., Wilkes, C. & Lipton, H. (2012). Advancing family-centred care in child and adolescent mental health: a critical review of the literature. *Healthcare Quarterly.* **15** (4), 64–75.

McCay, E., Cleverley, K., Danaher, A. & Mudachi, N. (2015). Collaborative partnerships: bridging the knowledge practice gap in client-centred care in mental health. *Journal of Mental Health Training, Education and Practice.* **10** (1), 51–60.

McEwan, B.S. & Seeman, T. (1999). Protective and damaging effects of mediators of stress. Elaborating and testing the concepts of allostasis and allostatic load. *Annals of the New York Academy of Sciences.* **896**, 30–47.

Manthorpe, J. & Samsi, K. (2016). Person-centered dementia care: current perspectives. *Clinical Interventions in Aging.* **11**, 1733–40.

Ministry of Health (1959). *The Welfare of Children in Hospital (The Platt Report).* London: HMSO.

National Institute for Health and Care Excellence (NICE) (2011). *Service user experience in adult mental health: improving the experience of care for people using adult NHS mental health services.* London: NICE.

National Institute for Health and Care Excellence (NICE) (2014). *Psychosis and schizophrenia in adults: prevention and management.* London: NICE.

National Institute for Health and Care Excellence (2016). *Dementia: supporting people with dementia and their carers in health and social care.* London: NICE.

Ontario Centre of Excellence for Child and Youth Mental Health (2017). *Developing a Family Engagement Model: Summary of the Literature.* Ottawa: Ontario Centre of Excellence for Child and Youth Mental Health.

Pharoah, F., Mari, J., Rathbone, J. & Wong, W. (2010). *Family intervention for schizophrenia.* Cochrane Database of Systematic Reviews.

Regan, K.M., Curtin, C. & Vorderer, L. (2006). Paradigm shifts in inpatient psychiatric care of children: approaching child- and family-centered care. *Journal of Child and Adolescent Psychiatric Nursing.* **19** (1), 29–40.

Robertson, J. & Robertson, J. (1971). Young children in brief separation: a fresh look. *Psychoanalytic Study of the Child.* **26**, 264–315.

Shields, L. (2010). Questioning family centred care. *Journal of Clinical Nursing.* doi: 10.1111/j.1365-2702.2010.03214.x.

Shields, L., Pratt, J., Davis, L.M. & Hunter, J. (2007). *Family-centred care for children in hospital.* Cochrane Database of Systematic Reviews. Issue 1. Art. No.: CD004811.

Shields, L., Zhou, H., Pratt, J., Taylor, M., Hunter, J. & Pascoe, E. (2012). *Family-centred care for hospitalised children aged 0-12 years.* Cochrane Database of Systematic Reviews. doi: 10.1002/14651858.CD004811.pub3.

Simpson, A., Hannigan, B., Coffey, M., Barlow, S., Cohen, R., Jones, A., Všetečková, J., Faulkner, A., Thornton, A. & Cartwright, M. (2016). Recovery-focused care planning and coordination in England and Wales: a cross-national mixed methods comparative case study. *BMC Psychiatry.* **16**, 147.

Simpson, A., Coffey, M., Hannigan, B., Barlow, S., Cohen, R., Jones, A., Faulkner, A., Thornton, A., Všetečková, J., Haddad, M. & Marlowe, K. (2017). Cross-national comparative case study of recovery-focused mental healthcare planning and coordination in acute inpatient mental health settings (COCAPP-A). *Health Services and Delivery Research.* **5**, 29.

Smith, L., Coleman, V. & Bradshaw, M. (2002). *Family Centred Care: Concept, Theory and Practice.* Hampshire: Palgrave.

Tallon, M.M., Kendall, G.E. & Snider, P.D. (2015). Rethinking family-centred care for the child and family in hospital. *Journal of Clinical Nursing.* **24**, 1426–35.

Wales Audit Office/Healthcare Inspectorate Wales (2009). *Services for Children and Young People with Emotional and Mental Health Needs.* Cardiff: Auditor General for Wales.

Chapter 2

Understanding and assessing the needs of families and carers

John Hyde

Introduction

Mental health problems do not just affect the individual – they also impact on their family, their wider social circle and their colleagues from work or education. Yet there is a tendency for mental health services to concentrate on the individual's condition without paying sufficient regard to the people who will be providing most care and support throughout that person's life.

This chapter will examine how families of people with mental health problems have been viewed historically. It will also consider how the individual's mental health problems affect the mental health, well-being and functioning of their family or carers.

The term 'family' will be used primarily, on the basis that much of the research within this area tends to focus on the family of a person with a mental health problem living within the household (Barrowclough 2005). But it should be noted that many of the findings may apply to other settings where the care of the person may be undertaken by the spouse, or other carers. For example, the concept of expressed emotion, as a measure of the emotional stress within a household was originally discovered through research on families of people with psychosis (Barrowclough & Tarrier 1992). However, this feature can be observed in other care environments, including staff within the healthcare sector (Barrowclough 2005).

This chapter will mainly look at working-age adults with mental health problems, whereas Chapters 4 and 10 will look specifically at the families of children and people with dementia. It should also be noted that some of the research and ideas on family and mental health (such as the issues of assessment, carer burden and the needs of families) have been derived from research with older adults, and then applied to the field of working-age adults (Lefley 2009).

Aims and learning outcomes

This chapter will look at the needs of families or carers of adults with mental health issues. Having read the chapter, the reader will:

- Understand carer burden
- Have a framework to determine the needs of a family member or carer.

The impact of caring for people with mental health problems

The overall rates of mental health problems in the population of England have been estimated at between 1 in 4 and 1 in 6 of the adult population (McManus et al. 2009, Bridges 2013). The high cost of providing ongoing care for people with disorders such as schizophrenia, bipolar disorder and dementia (through medication, outpatient and community care, benefit payments and hospitalisation and crisis intervention costs) mean that community care is not in fact a cheaper option than institutional care (Rogers & Pilgrim 2010).

Research on the long-term impact of mental health problems (such as schizophrenia and bipolar disorder) tends to reveal a great deal of variation in the course of the disorder and the outcome (Ciompi 1980, Carpenter & Kirkpatrick 1988, An der Heiden & Häfner 2015, Mason et al. 2018). Up to 80% of people with a disorder such as schizophrenia will relapse within the first two years after their initial diagnosis, and a similar number for those diagnosed with bipolar disorder (Stafford et al. 2013, Bengesser et al. 2013). The first three to five years are often characterised by higher rates of relapse, though this may stabilise over the long term (Mason et al. 2018). Additionally, this initial period is associated with the highest risk of attempted and completed suicide, with 40% of people with schizophrenia attempting suicide and 10% dying at their own hands (Hawton et al. 2005, Marshall & Rathbone 2011). When looking at ongoing symptoms of schizophrenia, there is a continuum, with approximately 30% experiencing some ongoing symptoms and about 20% experiencing significant ongoing symptoms of psychosis (Warner 2003). For the other 50%, there may be less severe symptoms or an absence of further psychotic episodes.

The research cited above has tended to focus on clinical measures (such as symptomatic changes in a disorder) and the treatment has therefore focused on the alleviation or removal of these symptoms rather than the more current idea of recovery. Much of the seminal research looking at working with families has focused primarily on symptom reduction. However, as the family-centred approach seeks to reduce stress and improve interpersonal communication within the household, this suggests that it can be effective in helping the person gain hope, purpose and meaning in their life (Thompson 2016).

The move to a more recovery-oriented mental health service has followed on from changes in the delivery of mental health care during the 1980s when the main emphasis in the UK switched from hospital-based care to community provision. A confluence of social and economic issues meant that large, outdated institutions were no longer providing appropriate care for people in a modern healthcare system, and such institutions were expensive to maintain (Rogers & Pilgrim 2001). With the closure of many old hospitals, greater emphasis was placed on communities and families supporting people with mental health problems (Rogers & Pilgrim 2010). This change in healthcare delivery has led to various problems for people with mental health problems and their families and these will be outlined below.

The traditional dominant model of mental health care has been and remains the medical model, which places the patient in the passive role of the recipient of care (Tyrer 2013). Treatments are aimed at reducing the symptoms of the illness and the impact the illness has on the person's life. Potentially, relatives are considered as peripheral to the person's treatment, or even allies to reinforce the medical model of care.

Over the years, the way healthcare professionals view the families has been tainted by theoretical viewpoints that have placed blame upon family members for the development of mental illness. The influential psychiatrist R.D. Laing proposed the idea that psychosis developed as a 'sane response to an insane world'. As he saw it, the family dynamics were a key part of this system, placing conflicting and competing demands on the child, so that 'insanity' was the 'logical' outcome (Laing 2010).

Others suggested that 'schizophrenogenic' mothers were the main people responsible for placing the child in this 'double-bind', and hence were the main causative factor when they developed mental health issues (Lefley 2009). The 'schizophrenogenic parent' was described as a person who was emotionally cold and rejecting, domineering and over-protective, unable to separate their own needs from those of the child. A child placed in this situation was said to develop delusions and thought disorder as a consequence of confusing and distorted messages from the parent. Such ideas were derived from the psychodynamic school of psychology. They were developed as explanatory theories, fitting in with a pre-existing theoretical framework, but lacked any basis in theoretical research and are now very rarely used (Lefley 2009).

More recently, there has been growing evidence implicating genetic factors in different types of mental illness, although the specific genes and pathways leading to particular disorders have not been identified (Owen et al. 2016). Some environmental factors, such as autumnal births, birth complications and maternal viruses, have also been implicated and are thought to account for a small but significant amount of variance (Craddock et al. 2009, Blows 2010).

In addition to these physical causes, some psychologists have suggested that abuse during childhood may be a significant factor in the development of a whole range of mental illnesses including psychosis (Bentall 2004). However, this does not suggest that abuse is causative in all cases, or indeed that the trauma has necessarily occurred within the family environment. Furthermore, as with genetic factors, the specific mechanisms of how such events lead to particular symptoms or diagnoses remain largely unknown.

Based on current evidence, we can conclude that the causes of mental health problems may come down to interactions between intrinsic factors, such as genes (Craddock et al. 2009, Blows 2010), and external factors, such as trauma (Wickham & Bentall 2016, Morrison 2009).

Expressed emotion

Although family relationships have not been identified as a definite cause of relapse in mental illness, they can have an impact on rates of relapse. This discovery followed the pioneering work of a team led by George Brown at the Medical Research Council Social Psychiatry Unit in the 1950s. They noted that there tended to be higher rates of relapse in individuals diagnosed with schizophrenia when they returned to live with their families. Further investigation, and interviews with the families, led to the identification of a measure of the level of stress within the home which they named 'expressed emotion' (Brown 1959, Amaresha & Venkatasubramanian 2012). This originally identified five factors, measured from a structured interview with the family members (see Table 2.1 below). Two of these factors (warmth and positive regard) were loosely correlated with positive outcomes.

And three factors (critical comments, hostility and emotional over-involvement) correlated with adverse outcomes.

Table 2.1: Expressed emotion *(Amaresha & Venkatasubramanian 2012)*

Expressed emotion	Description
Warmth	Expressed kindness, concern and empathy for the person
Positive regard	Statements expressing appreciation or support
Critical comments	Counting the number of personal criticisms of the person and their behaviour
Hostility	Expressions of anger or irritation, or attitudes expressing rejection of the person
Emotional over-involvement	Excessive self-sacrifice, over-protectiveness, and over-identification with the person

It should be noted that expressed emotion (EE) is not a trait or characteristic of a family; it is a measure of the stress within the household, originally proposed as a means of identifying areas of need within the family (Leff & Vaughn 1985). It is also noticeable that the positive features of EE (warmth and positive regard) have been featured less in the research on the family environment. This may be partly due to their lower correlation but it may also reflect models of care that tend to focus more on deficits, rather than developing and building on strengths.

Furthermore, as there is a correlation between the negative triad of EE and relapse rates, clinicians may no longer see the family as causing the illness but may consider the family responsible for relapse. However, it is not a simple cause and effect relationship. Expressed emotion may vary depending on the family's circumstances and the acuteness of the person's mental illness at the time (Birchwood & Cochrane 1990).

It is therefore important to consider the family's situation, which could have led to increased stress in the home environment. In most psychotic disorders, there will be a prolonged prodromal phase, with gradual changes in the person's behaviour and interpersonal relationships within the family. These changes may lead to difficulties in the family before any clear psychotic symptoms have emerged. The family may try to cope using the actions that have previously worked, or the strategies that appear at the time to be the best way of dealing with the person, based on what the family members believe is wrong with them.

When healthcare services become involved, families may or may not be given information about the person's diagnosis and treatment, and they may or may not be given advice and support. In this situation, the family members are likely to rely on their own lay beliefs about what is wrong with the person and what is the best course of action to take (Park et al. 2017). Meanwhile, some clinicians may assume that a family is high in EE because the family have caused the relapse, and the family may feel that they are being blamed by clinicians for the person's relapse.

To avoid these problems, the family should be seen not as a destructive influence on the person, but as people trying to cope with something they perhaps do not understand, using resources and ways of coping that may have worked in the past, but being frustrated by their inability to effect change in the person. The impact of the illness may have changed the person to such a degree that other family members feel estranged from them. On the other hand, family members may feel a desire to protect the person who they may see as fragile or vulnerable. In addition, they may feel that they are somehow responsible for causing the person's illness – a belief that could be reinforced by the discredited ideas discussed earlier, which tended to blame the family for the illness.

The earlier discussion would suggest that families rated as having high EE are the ones requiring help. However, NICE guidelines recommend that *all* families should be offered Family Intervention. Just because a family appears to be coping well, it should not be assumed that they would not wish for further help and input if it was offered (NICE 2014).

Illustrative case study

'Graham' is a 26-year-old man, who was admitted to hospital at 19 with his first episode of psychosis. He was treated with anti-psychotic medication and sent back home to live with his parents. Ongoing issues arising from his mental health problems included lack of motivation, poor hygiene and social isolation. Graham continued to take medication over the next few years and would attend outpatient appointments with his parents, but over time reduced and ceased contact with services.

At home Graham spent most of his time in his room playing computer games. His family would try and encourage him to eat with them and to attend social and family activities. However, on these occasions he would get into arguments with other family members, or his table manners would cause offence. The subjects of his conversation would sometimes lead to embarrassment with guests. Gradually over time the family tended to invite him out less to these social occasions, and Graham also preferred to avoid these situations. As the years went by, he spent more and more time on his own. His family found it easier to cope by separating a section of the house for Graham to use.

His parents continued to worry about how Graham's life was passing by and how he had no social outlet but were at a loss as to how to help him. Any attempts to encourage him into activities usually met with refusal. They felt guilty that they were not able to do more with Graham.

Reflection

- What is the role of healthcare practitioners with this family?
- Can you describe the relationship between the family's experience of stress and Graham's illness?

This case study highlights some issues regarding stress and family needs. It would not be surprising if an assessment of Graham's family suggested a low rating of EE. Graham and his parents have settled into a way of living that may reduce the instances of conflict but may not be satisfactory for all parties. Frustrations and concerns between family members may remain unexpressed and unresolved. New ways for the family to engage with each other are not being undertaken, as the family finds themselves in an impasse.

More generally, stress within the family may be a consequence of both the person's illness and the family's reactions, coping strategies and beliefs about the illness. Investigations into families identified as high in EE suggest that there is a tendency to be more rigid and inflexible in coping strategies, use avoidance as a way of coping and to perceive the behaviour of the person as a result of intrinsic personal factors rather than as a consequence of illness (Amaresha & Venkatasubramanian 2012, Barrowclough et al. 2005). The stress within the family can impact on the relapse rates for psychiatric conditions such as schizophrenia, bipolar disorder, depression and anxiety (Butzlaff & Hooley 1998) but it also affects the health and well-being of the family members, and this will be discussed in the next section.

Carer burden

Caring for someone who has extra needs because of mental or physical impairment can affect the well-being of the carer/s, or those who live in the same home environment. The following section will primarily concentrate on those caring for adults with mental health problems. There are some common features of being a carer, whether the person being cared for is an adult with a diagnosis of schizophrenia, an older adult with dementia, or a young person with an eating disorder. On the other hand, it should be noted that particular disorders at specific stages of a person's life do present their own unique challenges. Some reference will be made to these challenges, but it may be helpful to read other texts that go into more details on issues relating to caring for older adults, young people, or people with primary substance abuse problems.

In most instances, the role of carer falls upon family members (typically, the parents of adults and children, or the siblings of older adults). These family members will often be living in the same household as the person with mental health problems.

The term 'carer burden' is often used to describe the impact of caring for a person who is unwell upon the family members. This term tends to emphasise the negative aspects of the relationship, as a 'burden' is usually defined as an imposition upon a person or a load that is difficult to carry. Szmukler et al. (2003) suggest that the term 'experience of caregiving' does not carry the same pejorative connotations and allows for the positive aspects that people may experience when caring for another person. In this chapter both terms will be used, as 'carer burden' best encapsulates the negative impact of caring; and the more general term 'experience of caring' may better express the positive experiences, and strengths, that people may also find in caring.

Care burden is not that easy to describe or measure, for several reasons. Firstly, it may not be a stable phenomenon, as it may fluctuate, depending on the nature and severity of the person's illness at different times, and changes in the circumstances of the family members living with the person. Secondly, it can be defined and measured in different ways. It is commonly split into two areas: objective burden and subjective burden (Barrowclough 2005).

Therefore, when defining or measuring care burden, one needs to take into account: the situational factors; the ongoing experience of coping with mental health problems and other difficulties, by all family members; and the impact of events such as relapse, or behaviour resulting from the person's mental health problems. The burden of care can be split into objective burden and subjective burden (see Table 2.2).

Table 2.2: Carer burden (Baronet 1999)

Objective burden *The types of burden that can be observed and measured by an external agent, such as:*	Subjective burden *The types of burden that are intrinsic to the person, such as:*
• Time spent caring for the person • Financial impact • Transporting the person • Visiting the person in hospital • Diagnosis (of the person and family members) • Limitations on own activity.	• Perceived stress • Demands • Conflicts • Worry • Symptomatic, difficult or embarrassing behaviour.

These different aspects of burden have led to some difficulties in measurement, as there has been some variation in how it has been measured – by looking at either objective or subjective burden or a combination of the two. Although there is a correlation between objective and subjective burden, the process is mediated by intrinsic factors, such as the person's evaluation of their own illness and the impact it has upon them (Awad & Voruganti 2008). A parent with a child who has ongoing active symptoms, and who has left employment to look after the person (objective financial and time constraints), may perceive little subjective burden, if they do not see this as something that negatively impinges on their own life and well-being. On the other hand, a parent of a person who may have experienced a psychotic episode, but is largely symptom-free, may have ongoing worries about the illness, the possibility of relapse, and the long-term implications of the illness for the person and their family. In this situation, they may report a high degree of subjective burden.

Illustrative case study

To illustrate the complex issue of burden, look at the following example of a family living with a person with diagnosis of schizophrenia.

'James' is a 27-year-old man with a diagnosis of schizophrenia who lives at home with his parents. He has an ongoing belief that he is in contact with 'earth spirits', and that there are places in the world of special significance, which he wants to visit as they can enhance spiritual powers and help to heal the world. He also believes that herbs and hallucinogenic mushrooms help him to channel his spiritual self and communicate with the earth spirits. There have been times when he has left the family home to search for these special places, which has caused his parents a great deal of worry, as he has sometimes been missing for several days.

Generally, the family tolerate his unusual beliefs, are not critical and try to support him. He manages his daily activity most days, and he joins his family at mealtimes. Although he continues to express a desire to take hallucinogens, he has agreed with his family that he will limit their use and inform his family if he has taken them, so they can monitor him. He will also let them know in advance if he is planning to search out one of the sites and discuss this with his family.

After his most recent admission to hospital, it had been expected that he would return home. However, his parents had decided that they could no longer cope with his behaviour and the stress and worry of not knowing where he went. While James was in hospital, they found that they were able to relax more, and they realised the level of worry his behaviour had caused them over the years.

Reflection

- What do you see as the objective burdens for James and his family?
- What do you see as the subjective burdens for James and his family?
- If James were to return home, what support would be required?
- If James were not to return home, and was placed in alternative accommodation in the community, how might this affect the family?

As the above example illustrates, James's family may appear to be coping well with his illness and his behaviour. However, they may well find his use of drugs difficult to accept and be worried about his welfare if he is away from home for some time. Dealing with his fixation on spiritual ideas may also place strain on the family.

The effects of carer burden

Caring for a person with mental health problems can place a burden on the family, which can in turn impact on the mental health and well-being of the family. Mental illnesses such as schizophrenia and bipolar disorder often first emerge in the person's late teens to early twenties, and this may be a time when the person would be expected to become independent from the family, by going into employment or full-time education. As well as the impact of the illness there may be a significant adjustment in the family's expectations about what they hoped to be doing in later years. For carers of elderly relatives, these changes may occur during the period when the family's own children have recently left home, and they may have had expectations that did not include taking on the role of carer.

Based on the General Household Survey 2000 (cited in Barrowclough 2005), the majority of carers were looking after an elderly relative, usually a parent, and in most cases (67%) the person being cared for had mental health needs. For people diagnosed with a mental health problem (such as schizophrenia), 90% will return to live with their family. Although many may not experience further major mental health problems, many others will continue to be affected by their illness (Saunders 1999). The impact on the well-being of the carers is significant: 84% of carers report increased stress, and 55% feel more depressed. This is backed up by a study on carers of people with schizophrenia, reporting that 50% would meet the criteria for clinical depression. Additionally, 44% of carers report post-traumatic stress symptoms (Carers UK 2015).

A higher proportion of adults who take on the primary role of carer tend to be female and this accounts for the higher rates of symptoms of mental and physical illness in female relatives (Moller et *al.* 2009). However, other family members, such as siblings, may also find their mental and physical health partly affected by their experience of the person's mental health problems, as well as fear that they may be more liable to experience similar issues (Sin *et al.* 2015).

In conclusion, high levels of care burden may be partly due to the individual's subjective attitudes, beliefs and ways of coping with the person's illness, but they are also correlated with the level of external symptoms of illness, particularly the negative symptoms associated with schizophrenia.

Positive impact of caring

On the other hand, the experience of caring may not be experienced as uniformly negative. Some carers may enjoy the role of caring and may find that it helps them to develop new skills and resources. Having a positive experience of caring protects the carers from feeling burdened and thus also becomes a protective factor for the person receiving care (Watts & Hodgson 2016).

Other factors associated with positive coping are: social support for the carers, and support from services (both practical and emotional); an optimistic view of the person and of their own ability to cope; ability to distance themselves from the person's illness; and ability to use tension reduction strategies such as relaxation (Cotton *et al.* 2013).

General factors to consider when measuring expressed emotion

It should be noted that much of the original work on expressed emotion was conducted in the UK and was with predominantly white, British families. Across the world and within the UK, there is more cultural diversity since this original research took place. Family situations and cultural beliefs around mental illness and services may vary. Levels of EE may vary within different cultures and may be higher amongst white populations in countries such as the UK and lower in Mediterranean countries, Hispanic countries and Afro-Caribbean populations (Patel *et al.* 2014).

The Western model of the traditional nuclear family may not be typical of other cultures, which may include more members of the extended family in the home, providing additional family support. Religious beliefs may play a part in carer beliefs about illness, which can have both positive and negative aspects. A religious community may be a source of support for family, and they may find it helpful to see the person's illness framed positively in terms of spirituality, or helping the person find peace through prayer or medication. On the other hand, some religions may equate mental illness with sin, moral weakness or demonic possession (Cinnirella & Loewenthal 2011, Hartog & Gow 2005), which has the potential to increase stigma and burden. There may also be cultural beliefs around collectivist or individual ways of dealing with problems, as well as the view that people are fated to experience illness and disability.

Psychiatry itself has faced criticism for being ethnocentric, in terms of adopting a solely Western cultural perspective, and consequently experiencing difficulties with treating people from non-Western cultures. For instance, there are higher rates of detention of people from the Afro-Caribbean community and higher doses of medication. These factors may lead to higher levels of suspicion of healthcare professionals if people from particular cultures feel that services are likely to discriminate against them (Rogers & Pilgrim 2010). Such issues should be taken into account when considering who is best placed within the team to work with particular families, depending on their own background and culture.

In conclusion, mental health problems have wide-ranging effects, not just on the person, but also on their family. Time and resources can be taken up fulfilling the caring role. This can impact on social and economic aspects of family life, with changes in role, income and status. Although some may find benefits and strengths in the caring role, it is often considered a burden, and there may be risks to the physical and mental health of the carer.

Assessment tools used with families

The following list of assessment tools is not exhaustive but is intended to illustrate a variety of validated tools that can be used in the family setting. Some tools (such as the Relative Assessment Interview or the Knowledge About Schizophrenia Interview) take the form of semi-structured interviews, which can be used not only to gather knowledge about the family situation but also to structure a session.

It is important to be familiar with the assessment tools used in family work, and it is advisable to start by working with, and observing, a practitioner experienced in their use. In most instances, the assessment is conducted on a one-to-one basis with each family member and is not time limited. The assessment process can therefore take up a significant amount of time. However, the information gathered can be helpful for all concerned, in terms of clarifying areas of strength and need.

Most of the assessment tools in use in family intervention have been in use for several years and have not been superseded by more contemporary tools, which indicates their reliability. However, they could be criticised for tending to focus more on problems linked to the person's state, rather than the skills and strengths the family may possess (Rapp & Goscha 2006).

The process can combine informal assessment of information gathered through discussion with more formal assessment of information gathered using structured tools. Likewise, assessment can be holistic (looking at the whole family situation and the dynamic relationships between family members) as well as detailed, using specific tools that may examine particular aspects of the family. With any assessment, there is a need to engage with the family and discuss a rationale for working with them. In other words, what do the family members hope to gain by working collaboratively with services? This is an important part of the process of engagement. It develops from gaining a rapport and and it enables the practitioner to begin to understand the family's needs.

The main areas to consider when conducting an assessment are (Barrowclough & Tarrier 1992):

1. Relative's understanding of the illness and treatments
2. Distress to relative caused by the symptoms and situations
3. Coping strategies to deal with symptoms and behaviours
4. The impact of the illness on the family members – objective burden
5. The relationship between the carer and the person with mental health problems
6. Areas of strengths, such as coping strategies and social support.

Relative Assessment Interview (RAI)

The Relative Assessment Interview is a semi-structured interview and the interviewer should be familiar with the tool. As with most family work, it should ideally be facilitated by two practitioners. In the first instance, it would be useful to train in its use and work alongside an experienced practitioner to gain familiarity. This will also help to make the process of completing the assessment more relaxed and informal (Barrowclough & Tarrier 1992). Ideally it should be completed with each family member. It is possible to complete it with a whole family group, but this should be avoided where possible – the risks being that not everyone's voice is heard and that some family members may feel they are being singled out for criticism by other members of the family.

Completing assessments such as this can also elicit strong emotions as people recall and discuss distressing events and behaviours. The process of completing the assessment should therefore not be time limited; nor should completion of the assessment be prioritised over the family's needs. Time may have to be allowed for the family to discuss these issues (Smith et al. 2007). Furthermore, as the RAI will take some time to complete, it may be useful to take breaks, or to complete it over more than one session – although ideally this will still be within a short time frame (e.g. within a week).

The RAI is a good starting point, as it gives an overall view of the family members, their viewpoints and their concerns, before the practitioner moves on to using more specific tools.

The RAI covers the following five areas with prompts and questions to discuss in more detail:

1. Background information
2. Psychiatric history
3. Current problems/symptoms
4. Relationship between family members
5. General information about the relative.

The full transcript for this assessment and all the assessment tools discussed is available in *Families of Schizophrenic Patients* (Barrowclough & Tarrier 1992).

KGV symptom scale

This scale can be used with the person who has been diagnosed with a mental illness and it is a useful tool to help the practitioner begin to gain an understanding of any ongoing symptoms from the person's perspective (see Table 2.3 on page 26).

In the first part of the scale there are specific questions to ask to elicit symptoms, and additional suggested prompt questions to enable the person to elaborate on their answer. Each area can be scored, as the questionnaire was originally devised as a research tool. It is advisable to be trained in the scoring of the scale to gain a level of consistency with other users. However, the scale can be used solely for the purpose of gaining an understanding of the individual being assessed.

Table 2.3: Areas of assessment in the KGV symptom scale *(Krawiecka et al. 1977)*
This is a semi-structured interview which looks at the following areas.

Elicited by questioning	Elicited by observation:
• Mood (anxiety, depressed mood, elevated mood) • Suicidal ideation and behaviour • Hallucinations • Delusions.	• Affect (flattened or incongruous) • Overactivity • Psychomotor retardation • Abnormal speech, poverty of speech • Abnormal movements • Accuracy of assessment.

Based on experience of using this tool, it can help reveal more information than expected about people's thoughts and feelings, even in people you may have known for some time. It can also be beneficial for the person to talk about some issues that have often been overlooked, ignored or dismissed. The KGV assessment can be lengthy, and it may touch on sensitive topics such as suicidal ideation, so it requires careful questioning and management, when high-risk issues are revealed.

Family Questionnaire (FQ)

Unlike the RAI, which provides a great deal of qualitative data on the family, the FQ is a more formal structured scoring sheet and should ideally be given to all carers who are willing to participate in any form of family intervention.

This tool asks a series of 49 questions such as:

- Talks to himself or imaginary persons.

The relative is then asked to rate how often this happens, from 1 (never) to 5 (always).

Then the relative rates, on a scale of 1 to 5, how much this bothers them. Finally, on a scale of 1 to 5, they rate their ability to cope with the behaviour.

The FQ ratings should look at recent behaviour, rather than historical behaviour. This tool can be used to identify those areas of concern which the relative finds distressing and difficult to cope with, in order to highlight areas to focus on when helping the family.

The FQ should be completed individually and can be completed by the person on their own or during a session. If you ask the person to complete it alone, it is valuable to go through the first few questions during a session to check that the person fully understands the process of completing the form.

Social Functioning Scale (SFS)

This is a structured scale and, as the title suggests, it focuses specifically on social functioning. It examines six areas of social and vocational functioning:

1. Social withdrawal

2. Interpersonal functioning
3. Prosocial activities
4. Recreation
5. Level of independence
6. Employment.

Each area is scored and can be compared with the population mean, using the chart that comes with the scale.

Knowledge About Schizophrenia Interview (KASI)

The KASI is also a semi-structured interview, which is used to determine the relative's knowledge and understanding of the person's illness. In addition to questions that can elicit discussion, there are specific questions that can be rated. You can use the questionnaire to guide discussion and not use the scoring. Alternatively, you can use the scoring to identify areas to work on, to quantify the extent of the relative's knowledge and to provide a baseline for further retest scores after any interventions.

The KASI looks at six areas of functioning:

1. Diagnosis
2. Symptomatology
3. Medication
4. Course and prognosis
5. Management.

Although the title indicates that this tool can only be used to assess families of people with schizophrenia, the word 'schizophrenia' can simply be changed to 'psychosis' to adapt the questions to a wider range of conditions. It should be noted that the validity of the scoring may be affected, but this may not be such an important issue if you are using it in routine practice rather than as part of a research programme.

Other tools

The above tools are intended to be used when working with families, but there are other tools that you may wish to use, to gain further understanding of the family's health and wellbeing (e.g. General Health Questionnaire), as well as understanding of treatment and side effects (e.g. the Drug Attitude Inventory or the Liverpool University Side Effects Rating Scale).

A number of assessment tools are used in family work and assessment may be time-consuming, but it is key to gaining a clear understanding of the family. The process itself can also be illuminating for the family and may provide insights and benefits before any formal intervention has begun. The quality of the information gained in the assessment will provide a firm basis for the work that follows.

Reflection

If you were working with a family where an adult had a mental health issue, which assessment tool/s do you think would be most helpful in determining the needs of the family or carer?

Conclusion

Historically, families and carers of people with mental health problems have too often either been considered as the cause of the person's mental health problem, or have not been sufficiently engaged by services in the care and treatment of the person (Lefley 2009). As services continue to move towards a model of treatment within the community, there is an ever-greater need for healthcare professionals to engage with the families. There is a moral imperative to give families information about the illness of the person they will be looking after, and there is also empirical evidence to show that working with families to increase knowledge, and reduce their level of stress, reduces the chances of the individual relapsing (with the huge social and economic consequences relapse brings).

The first step in helping the families is to gain an understanding of their needs. A thorough, systematic assessment can provide several benefits. It can enable the practitioner to gain the information needed to help the family (as part of the process of engagement); it can also allow the family to give voice to their experiences and concerns.

References

Amaresha, A. C. & Venkatasubramanian, G. (2012). Expressed emotion in schizophrenia: an overview. *Indian Journal of Psychological Medicine.* **34**, 12–20.

An der Heiden, W. & Häfner, H. (2015). Investigating the long-term course of schizophrenia by sequence analysis. *Psychiatry Research.* **228**, 551–59.

Awad, A.G. & Voruganti, L.N.P. (2008). The burden of schizophrenia on caregivers: A review. *PharmacoEconomics.* **26**, 149–62.

Baronet, T.A.M. (1999). Factors associated with caregiver burden in mental illness: a critical review of the research literature. *Clinical Psychology Review.* **19**, 819–41.

Barrowclough, C. (2005). 'Families of People with Schizophrenia' In: N. Sartorius, J. Leff, J.J. Lopez-Ibor, M. Maj, M. & A. Okasha (eds) *Families and Mental Disorder: From Burden to Empowerment.* Chichester: John Wiley & Sons.

Barrowclough, C. & Tarrier, N. (1992). *Families of Schizophrenic Patients: Cognitive Behavioural Intervention.* Cheltenham: Stanley Thornes.

Barrowclough, C., Ward, J., Wearden, A., Gregg, L. (2005). Expressed emotion and attributions in relatives of schizophrenia patients with and without substance misuse. *Social Psychiatry and Psychiatric Epidemiology.* **40**, 884–91.

Bengesser, S.A., Reininghaus, B., Birner, A., Lackner, N., Kapfhammer, H.P. & Reininghaus, E.Z. (2013). Bipolar disorder and compliance. *Fortschritte der Neurologie Psychiatrie.* **81**, 398–400.

Bentall, R.P. (2004). *Madness Explained: Psychosis and Human Nature.* London: Penguin Adult.

Birchwood, M. & Cochrane, R. (1990). Families coping with schizophrenia: coping styles, their origins and correlates. *Psychological Medicine.* **20**, 857–65.

Blows, W.T. (2010). *The Biological Basis of Mental Health Nursing.* London: Taylor & Francis.

Bridges, S. (2013). 'Mental health problems' In: R. Craig & J. Mindell (eds) *Health Survey for England 2014: Health, social care and lifestyles.* Leeds: The Health and Social Care Information Centre.

Brown, G.W. (1959). Experiences of discharged chronic schizophrenic patients in various types of living group. *The Milbank Memorial Fund Quarterly.* **37**, 105–31.

Butzlaff, R.L. & Hooley, J.M. (1998). Expressed emotion and psychiatric relapse: A meta-analysis. *Archives of General Psychiatry.* **55**, 547–52.

Carers UK (2015). *State of Caring 2015.* London: Carers UK.

Carpenter, J.W.T. & Kirkpatrick, B. (1988). The heterogeneity of the long-term course of schizophrenia. *Schizophrenia Bulletin.* **14**, 645–52.

Cinnirella, M. & Lowenthal, K.M. (2011). Religious and ethnic group influences on beliefs about mental illness: A qualitative interview study. *British Journal of Medical Psychology.* **72**, 505–24.

Ciompi, L. (1980). Catamnestic long-term study on the course of life and aging of schizophrenics. *Schizophrenia Bulletin.* **6**, 606–18.

Cotton, S.M., McCann, T.V., Gleeson, J.F., Crisp, K., Murphy, B.P. & Lubman, D.I. (2013). Coping strategies in carers of young people with a first episode of psychosis. *Schizophrenia Research.* **146**, 118–24.

Craddock N., O'Donovan M.C. & Owen M.J. (2009). Psychosis genetics: modelling the relationship between schizophrenia, bipolar disorder, and mixed (or 'schizoaffective') psychoses. *Schizophrenia Bulletin.* **35**, 482–90.

Hartog, K. & Gow K.M. (2005). Religious attributions pertaining to the causes and cures of mental illness. *Mental Health, Religion & Culture.* **8**, 263–76.

Hawton K., Sutton, L., Haw C., Sinclair, J. & Deeks, J.J. (2005). Schizophrenia and suicide: systematic review of risk factors. *The British Journal of Psychiatry.* **187**, 9–20.

Krawiecka M., Goldberg D. & Vaughan M. (1977). A standardized psychiatric assessment scale for rating chronic psychotic patients. *Acta Psychiatrica Scandinavica.* **55**, 299–308.

Laing, R. (2010). *The Divided Self: An Existential Study in Sanity and Madness.* London: Penguin Books Limited.

Leff, J.P. & Vaughn, C. (1985). *Expressed Emotion in Families: its Significance for Mental Illness.* New York: Guilford Press.

Lefley, H.P. (2009). *Family Psychoeducation for Serious Mental Illness.* Oxford:Oxford University Press.

Marshall, M. & Rathbone, J. (2011). *Early intervention for psychosis.* Cochrane Database of Systematic Reviews.

Mason, P., Harrison, G., Glazebrook, C., Medley, I. & Croudacce, T. (2018). The course of schizophrenia over 13 years: a report from the International Study on Schizophrenia (ISoS) coordinated by the World Health Organization. *British Journal of Psychiatry.* **169**, 580–86.

McManus, S. Meltzer, H., Brugha, T. & Bebbington P. (eds) (2009). Adult Psychiatric Morbidity in England, 2007: Results of a Household Survey: The NHS Information Centre for Health and Social Care.

Moller, T., Gudde, C.B., Folden, G.E. & Linaker, O.M. (2009). The experience of caring in relatives to patients with serious mental illness: gender differences, health and functioning. *Scandinavian Journal of Caring Sciences.* **23**, 153–60.

Morrison, A.P. (2009). A cognitive behavioural perspective on the relationship between childhood trauma and psychosis. *Epidemiologia e psichiatria sociale.* **18**, 294–98.

National Institute for Health and Care Excellence (NICE) (2014). *Psychosis and schizophrenia in adults: treatment and management.* London: National Institute for Health and Care Excellence.

Owen M.J., Sawa, A. & Mortensen, P.B. (2016). Schizophrenia. *The Lancet.* **388**, 86–97.

Park, S., Lee, M., Furnham, A., Jeon, M, Ko, Y.-M. (2017). Lay beliefs about the causes and cures of schizophrenia. *International Journal of Social Psychiatry.* **63**, 518–24.

Patel, M., Chawla, R., Krynicki, C.R., Rankin, P. & Upthegrove, R. (2014). Health beliefs and carer burden in first episode psychosis. *Behavioural Medicine and Primary Care Psychiatry.* **14**, 171.

Rapp, C.A. & Goscha, R.J. (2006). *The Strengths Model: Case Management with People with Psychiatric Disabilities.* Oxford University Press.

Rogers, A. & Pilgrim, D. (2001). *Mental Health Policy in Britain.* Basingstoke: Palgrave Macmillan.

Rogers, A. & Pilgrim, D. (2010). *A Sociology of Mental Health and Illness.* Maidenhead: McGraw-Hill Education.

Saunders, J.C. (1999). Family functioning in families providing care for a family member with schizophrenia. *Issues in Mental Health Nursing.* **20**, 95–113.

Simpson, S., Barnes, E., Griffiths, E., Hood, K., Cohen, D., Craddock, N., Jones, I. & Smith, D. J. (2009). The Bipolar Interactive Psychoeducation (BIPED) study: trial design and protocol. *BMC Psychiatry.* **9**, 50.

Sin, J., Jordan, C. D., Barley, E. A., Henderson, C. & Norman, I. (2015). *Psychoeducation for siblings of people with severe mental illness.* Cochrane Database Systematic Review. CD010540.

Smith, G., Higgs, A. & Gregory, K. (2007). *An Integrated Approach to Family Work for Psychosis: A Manual for Family Workers.* London: Jessica Kingsley Publishers.

Stafford, M.R., Jackson, H., Mayo-Wilson, E., Morrison, A.P. & Kendall, T. (2013). Early interventions to prevent psychosis: systematic review and meta-analysis. *British Medical Journal.* **346** doi: https://doi.org/10.1136/bmj.f185 (last accessed 30.9.2019).

Szmukler, G., Kuipers, E., Joyce, J., Harris, T., Leese, M., Maphosa, W. & Staples, E. (2003). An exploratory randomised controlled trial of a support programme for carers of patients with a psychosis. *Social Psychiatry and Psychiatric Epidemiology.* **38**, 411–18.

Thompson F. (2016). 'The Mental Health Nurse and Recovery'. In: S. Trenoweth (ed.) *Promoting Recovery in Mental Health Nursing.* London: SAGE Publications.

Tyrer, P. (2013). *Models for Mental Disorder.* Chichester: Wiley.

Warner, R. (2003). *Recovery from Schizophrenia: Psychiatry and Political Economy.* London: Taylor & Francis.

Watts, L. & Hodgson, D. (2016). Assessing the needs of carers of people with mental illness: lessons from a collaborative study. *Practice.* **28**, 235–52.

Wickham, S. & Bentall, R. (2016). Are specific early-life adversities associated with specific symptoms of psychosis? a patient study considering just world beliefs as a mediator. *The Journal of Nervous and Mental Disease.*

Chapter 3

Working with families affected by psychosis

Alicia Stringfellow

Introduction

This chapter will highlight the theoretical basis for family intervention when working with individuals with psychosis. It will also provide a step-by-step explanation of some of the therapeutic skills practitioners can utilise to support service users and their families. Psycho-education, problem-solving and goal setting will all be discussed in the context of family working, and consideration will be given to practitioner supervision when working with families. The aim is to share an appreciation of working with families of individuals with psychosis, identifying the purpose, goals and benefits of this work; discussing a range of skills to facilitate specific family intervention techniques; and explaining the value of supervision for this work.

Background

Psychosis is a term used to describe a range of serious mental health conditions, such as schizophrenia, bipolar disorder, schizo-affective disorder and drug-induced psychosis. It is characterised by a range of symptoms that alter a person's perception, thoughts, mood and behaviour. Psychosis can be severe and debilitating, characterised by profound disruptions in thinking, affecting language, perception, and the sense of self (American Psychiatric Association 2013). Psychosis typically begins in late adolescence or early adulthood and may include hallucinations, delusions, disorganised speech and thought disorder. A range of negative symptoms that impact on social functioning may also develop, including alogia (lack of speech), anhedonia (the inability to experience pleasure), lack of volition and flattened affect. Each person with a psychotic disorder will have a unique combination of symptoms and experience (NICE 2014).

The impact of psychosis, on people, their carers, family members, healthcare services and society in general, is significant; and due to the range of health and social needs associated with the illness, the financial cost is high (Schizophrenia Commission 2012).

In recent years there has been an acknowledgment of the importance of early recognition of the signs and symptoms of psychosis, with a shift from a traditional medical model to a bio-psychosocial model that focuses on prevention, early detection and intervention (Birchwood *et al.* 2013, Morrison *et al.* 2012, Addington *et al.* 2011). For those with psychotic symptoms, early intervention is crucial to improving outcomes and early treatment of psychosis is one of the most significant developments in mental health care since the beginning of community care (Birchwood *et al.* 2013). Nevertheless, a significant number of people with a more established psychotic illness find themselves on the fringes of society and many of them are primarily cared for and supported by family members. It is estimated that families who provide care for those affected by psychosis significantly reduce annual public spending; yet those with psychosis, their families and carers continue to report a lack of best practice interventions and a lack of involvement in care (Schizophrenia Commission 2012).

Families can find witnessing and living with the day-to-day fluctuations, symptoms and behaviours associated with psychosis confusing, frustrating and frightening (Marder & Freedman 2014). Most are ill-prepared to cope and have little knowledge of the condition. They may also be frustrated by difficulties in accessing help and navigating a complex healthcare system (Tuck *et al.* 1997, Pitschel-Walz *et al.* 2001, Coker *et al.* 2016). In addition, they may find that they are subject to unhelpful and stigmatising stereotypes (Connor *et al.* 2016).

Alongside medication, a range of interventions are recommended for those with psychosis and their families and carers, including psycho-education programmes, communication skills training, problem-solving and relapse prevention (Falloon *et al.* 2004, NICE 2014). Despite these recommendations, however, family intervention is not routinely offered to family members by mental health services and practitioners (Michie *et al.* 2007, Berry & Hadock 2008, Hackman & Dixon 2008, All Party Parliamentary Group on Mental Health 2010). This may suggest that the burden associated with caring for a loved one with psychosis, and the resulting interactions within the family, are still significant factors in relation to relapse.

Working in collaboration with service users and their families, family intervention offers an approach that builds on the strengths within the family, explores solutions to the problems they face as a result of the illness, and enables the practitioner to facilitate and support the family to tackle any difficulties. The ultimate aim of working with families of those with psychosis is to promote understanding of, and recovery from, psychosis and to improve the individual's social functioning and independence (Stringfellow 2016).

Aims and learning outcomes

This chapter aims to highlight the theoretical basis for family intervention for individuals with psychosis and explain some of the therapeutic skills practitioners can utilise to support service users and their families. Having completed the chapter, the reader will have:

- An understanding of psycho-education and problem-solving as processes
- An overview of how relapse prevention techniques can be used with families
- An understanding of the importance of practitioner supervision when working with families.

Psycho-education

Family members may avoid discussing family issues with the service user for fear of escalating uncomfortable situations and worsening the symptoms of the illness. They may also avoid discussing the situation with people outside the family unit for fear of stigma and embarrassment. Mental health practitioners may feel uncomfortable communicating with family members, perhaps due to issues around confidentiality or because they are not adequately equipped with the skills and confidence to discuss and address challenging questions or negative views from family members in relation to past experiences or inadequate service delivery. Additionally, the practitioner may not know or fully understand what is wrong, and may not want to confuse or burden family members further. Furthermore, inexperience and not wanting to upset family members may hinder effective information sharing. Therefore, any information relating to the psychotic illness (for example, regarding signs, symptoms, what may be helpful or unhelpful, or what to do in a crisis) may not have been communicated clearly, despite families consistently asking for information and advice on how to approach some of the difficult situations they face.

Generally, family members do not expect clear-cut answers to questions but want to be given up-to-date, relevant and appropriate information; they usually welcome the opportunity to discuss practical ways of addressing difficulties and managing stress. When working with families, it is important for mental health practitioners to share information and gain understanding in a two-way process with both service users and family members. This enables the practitioner to make sense of the issues faced by the family in the context of the illness and to meet their needs more effectively. It also helps the service user make sense of their experience and assists the family in gaining knowledge and a greater understanding of the illness and the unique signs and symptoms they experience and observe.

When commencing psycho-education sessions, the service user and their family members should be viewed as the experts, as their experience of psychosis will be unique to them. The mental health practitioner will have gained knowledge more broadly in regard to the illness but both these sources of knowledge should be respected and acknowledged within a collaborative therapeutic relationship. Sharing information and promoting shared decision-making in this way is congruent with the principles of co-production whereby service users, their families and carers are equal partners in all aspects of their care.

Attention should also be paid to the environment in which the information is communicated. This should ideally be a quiet, private space, away from distractions and interruptions. Generally, buildings that house mental health services should be avoided, as the family may view the mental health practitioner as the expert in such an environment. This perceived imbalance of power may make it more difficult to convey the message that they, as service users and family members, are the experts and that their lived experience is valued. Sharing information in the family home tends to be more beneficial, as family members are likely to feel more at ease, less distracted and more in control.

A rationale for information sharing should be provided by the mental health practitioner, and the benefits of gaining further knowledge and understanding of the illness should be highlighted. A clear explanation should be given of how this enhanced knowledge and understanding may help them manage the situation more effectively.

Setting an agenda with the family for the psycho-education session may be beneficial, as it can provide an outline of what is going to be covered in the session and also enable the person affected by psychosis and family members to prioritise different topics and suggest the order in which they would like the information to be communicated. The sessions should be time limited and the family members should feel able to ask questions throughout the session as well as at the end. Short, frequent sessions are often more beneficial than longer ones, and consideration will need to be given to each family member's concentration levels and their ability to process information.

Leaving relevant literature with the family is helpful and allows them to refer to it again at their leisure between sessions. The mental health practitioner should also be ready to signpost the family to other relevant, appropriate sources of information, should the family request it, and have a list of websites and telephone numbers available. Information should be clear, concise and jargon-free, and care should be taken to ensure the the information is provided in a user-friendly form that is appropriate to the educational level of all concerned. A stepwise prompt for preparing for family work sessions is given in Table 3.1 below.

The information shared may have a significant emotional impact on some or all family members; each will have their own personal experience and views about their current situation; about the illness and about mental health services and support. They may have accessed inappropriate or inaccurate information in the past from a variety of sources. The mental health practitioner must therefore ensure that the information communicated is relevant, evidence-based and appropriate to the family's requirements.

Table 3.1: Preparation for psycho-education sessions with a family

● Take time to prepare for the session. An understanding of the needs of the family will help determine the information to be shared.
● Ensure the material is appropriate for the family. Familiarise yourself with any relevant pre-prepared material, information from websites, videos, etc.
● Try to anticipate any possible questions relating to the material used.
● Recognise that the session may raise some questions that cannot be answered (such as Why me? Why us?). Exploring these issues within a recovery-focused framework can be beneficial.
● Maintain a calm, non-threatening environment. Any hostile or accusatory exchanges should be stopped, as these will impede learning and may result in family members disengaging.
● Leave relevant information with family members at the end of the session so they can refer to it in their own time.

Confidentiality

Complex legal, professional and ethical issues relating to confidentiality may be a barrier to fully engaging with family members and may even be a reason to avoid working fully in this way.

It is therefore worth taking time within the psycho-education sessions to explore the issue of confidentiality with service users and their family members in an open and transparent way, highlighting what can and cannot be shared. This can help inform ground rules for the psycho-education sessions. Doing this will not only allow the mental health practitioner to feel more comfortable when discussing pertinent information but it will also enhance family members' understanding of how they can work together to solve problems and negotiate solutions without breaching service user confidentiality.

Problem-solving and goal setting
Problem-solving

An important part of working with families of those with psychosis is helping them develop effective problem-solving. This is a skill that the mental health practitioner can introduce either in response to a specific problem or when the family report more general difficulties with their current situation. However, using the term 'problem-solving' may cause the family to view themselves as 'a problem family' so it is important to use terminology that family members feel comfortable with. Suggesting that this is a skill that can facilitate planning, and that it can help them address everyday issues that occur within lots of families, may help the family to view the skill more positively. Likewise, identifying goals (rather than problems) helps both the practitioner and family members to tackle issues collaboratively. Identifying these goals is an important first step. For example, 'the dog never gets walked' becomes 'how to ensure the dog gets walked'. Reframing issues in this way not only enables people to approach problems more positively but it can also encourage all family members to look for solutions to their current difficulties.

Previous knowledge of the service user and individual family members will help the mental health practitioner recognise and verbalise the existing strengths within the family and their ability to problem-solve and set goals. Falloon *et al.* (2004) suggest a six-step problem-solving approach when working with families of those with psychosis and this approach is now part of specific behavioural family intervention programmes for this client group. Whilst learning and practising the technique, it is important for the mental health practitioner to stress that the family should initially focus on reasonably straightforward problems, as this will help the family to avoid arguments or conflict within the session.

Here is a sample dialogue:

MH professional: I would like to introduce a process called problem-solving that may be useful to you as a family to help you agree on solutions to some of your everyday problems. I have observed that you are sometimes able to discuss issues affecting you all and reach solutions – for example, the time when the car wouldn't start when you needed to get Liz to her hospital appointment. There are other times though, from what you have told me previously, when some of the day-to-day problems you encounter can lead to arguments and ill-feeling and you don't always communicate with each other to solve these. Would that be a true reflection of family life here?

Allow all family members to comment.

MH professional: How do you think it would help you as a family if you were able to solve problems in a more constructive and positive way?

Allow all family members to comment.

MH professional: Sometimes it can be helpful to work on solving problems together as a family step-by-step but this can take practice. The more families meet to discuss problems, the more able they become to sort these out without argument and ill-feeling. Whilst sometimes there is no perfect answer, this collaborative approach appears to help.

The MH professional then introduces the problem-solving worksheet to family members (see Table 3.2 below).

Table 3.2: Six-step problem-solving worksheet *(adapted from Falloon et al. (2004)*

STEP 1: WHAT IS THE PROBLEM OR GOAL? Talk about the problem or goal, listen carefully, ask questions, get everybody's opinion. Then write down exactly what the problem or goal is. ....
STEP 2: LIST ALL POSSIBLE SOLUTIONS Put down all ideas, even if you are not sure they will work. Get everybody to come up with at least one possible solution. List the solutions without discussion at this stage. 1. .... 2. .... 3. ....
STEP 3: DISCUSS EACH POSSIBLE SOLUTION Quickly go down the list of possible solutions and discuss the main advantages and disadvantages of each one.
STEP 4: CHOOSE THE BEST SOLUTION Choose the solution that can be carried out most easily to deal with the problem or achieve the goal.
STEP 5: PLAN HOW TO CARRY OUT THE BEST SOLUTION Discuss the resources needed and the major pitfalls to overcome. Practise difficult steps. Plan time for review. 1. .... 2. ....
STEP 6: REVIEW RESULTS Focus on achievement first – what worked well? Review plan. Make any changes that are necessary.

Having introduced the six-step approach, the mental health practitioner should instruct the family to practise the skill and provide feedback on their performance, highlighting the strengths observed within the family.

> **MH professional:** I particularly like the way you were all able to offer some potential solutions to walking the dog more regularly and were able to quickly discuss these potential solutions and choose the best result for you all.

The practitioner should encourage between-session practice and revisit the family's progress with problem-solving each time they meet. This will help the family develop their problem-solving skills and slowly work up to tackling some of the bigger issues they face.

References

Addington, J., Cornblatt, B., Cadenhead, K., Cannon, T., McGlashan, T., Perkins, D., Seidman, L., Tsuang, M., Walker, E., Woods, S. & Heinssen, R. (2011). At clinical high risk for psychosis: outcome for nonconverters. *American Journal of Psychiatry.* **168** (8), 800–805.

All Party Parliamentary Group on Mental Health (2010). *Health and Social Care Reform: making it work for mental health.*

American Psychiatric Association (2013). *Diagnostic and Statistical Manual of Mental Disorders.* Washington: American Psychiatric Association.

Berry, K. & Haddock, G. (2008). The implementation of the NICE guidelines for schizophrenia: Barriers to the implementation of psychological interventions and recommendations for the future. *Psychology and Psychotherapy: Theory, Research and Practice.* **81**, 419–36.

Birchwood, M., Connor, C., Lester, H., Patterson, P., Freemantle, N., Marshall, M., Fowler, D., Lewis, S., Jones, P., Amos, T. & Everard, L. (2013). Reducing duration of untreated psychosis: care pathways to early intervention in psychosis services. *The British Journal of Psychiatry.* **203** (1), 58–64.

Coker, F., Williams, A., Hayes, L., Hamann, J. & Harvey, C. (2016). Exploring the needs of diverse consumers experiencing mental illness and their families through family psychoeducation. *Journal of Mental Health.* **25** (3), 197–203.

Connor, C., Greenfield, S., Lester, H., Channa, S., Palmer, C., Barker, C., Lavis, A. & Birchwood, M. (2016). Seeking help for first-episode psychosis: a family narrative. *Early Intervention in Psychiatry.* **10** (4), 334–45.

Falloon, I., Montero, I., Sungur, M., Mastroeni, A., Malm, U., Economou, M., Grawe R., Harangozo, J., Mizuno, M., Murakami, M. & Hager, B. (2004). Implementation of evidence-based treatment for schizophrenic disorders: two-year outcome of an international field trial of optimal treatment. *World Psychiatry.* **3** (2), 104.

Hackman, A. & Dixon, L. (2008). Issues in family services for persons with schizophrenia: evidenced based interventions and future directions. *Psychiatric Times.* **25** (3), 45–52.

Marder, S. & Freedman, R. (2014). Learning from people with schizophrenia. *Schizophrenia Bulletin.* **40** (6), 1185–86.

Michie, S., Pilling, S., Garety, P., Whitty, P., Eccles, M., Johnston, M. & Simmons, J. (2007). Difficulties implementing a mental health guideline: an exploratory investigation using psychological theory. Implementation. *Science.* **2** (1), 8.

Morrison, A., French, P., Stewart, S., Birchwood, M., Fowler, D., Gumley, A., Jones, P., Bentall, R., Lewis, S., Murray, G. & Patterson, P. (2012) Early detection and intervention evaluation for people at risk of psychosis: multisite randomised controlled trial. *British Medical Journal.* **344**, e2233.

National Institute for Health and Care Excellence (NICE) (2014). *Psychosis and schizophrenia in adults: treatment and management.* London: National Collaborating Centre for Mental Health.

Pitschel-Walz, P., Leucht, S., Baum, J., Kissling, W. & Engel, R. (2001) The effect of family intervention on relapse and re-hospitalization in schizophrenia – a meta-analysis. *Schizophrenia Bulletin.* **27** (1), 73–92.

Schizophrenia Commission (2012). *The Abandoned Illness.* https://mentalhealthpartnerships.com/resource/the-abandoned-illness-a-report-by-the-schizophrenia-commission/ (Last accessed 2.8.2019).

Stringfellow, A. (2016). 'Family Intervention in Psychosis.' In: N. Evans & B. Hannigan (eds) *Therapeutic Skills for Mental Health Nurses.* London: Open University Press. 204–17

Tuck, I., du Mont, P., Evans, G. & Shupe, J. (1997). The experience of caring for an adult child with schizophrenia. *Archives of Psychiatric Nursing.* **11** (3), 118–25.

Chapter 4

Parents with mental health issues – thinking about the whole family

Nicola Evans

Introduction

Throughout this book there are chapters that discuss family approaches related mainly to adults with mental health issues in a range of settings (such as Chapter 7, on forensic services) or adults with specific mental health conditions (such as Chapter 3, on psychosis). This chapter, in contrast, is an opportunity to think more generally about the adults who access our range of mental health services who also happen to be parents.

When I reflect upon my own clinical experience and have conversations with colleagues currently in clinical practice, I notice that mental health services are often centred on the individual person accessing the service. Occasionally, questions are asked about family involvement or structure, and this line of inquiry is pursued in services that offer family interventions. However, perhaps the issues relating to being a parent are commonly missed, or merely touched upon in initial assessments. Parenting is such an important part of people's lives that it needs proper attention and consideration, so this chapter offers ways of thinking about parents who access mental health services.

We know that around 1 in 4 people in the UK experience a mental health issue, so we must assume that a reasonable proportion of these people are also parents. It is estimated that possibly 68% of women and 57% of men with a mental illness are parents (Royal College of Psychiatrists 2014) and up to 66% of people with a serious mental illness may be living with one or more children under the age of 18 years (Bee *et al.* 2014). However, mental health services in the UK are generally designed within an age-defined structure. Children and young people access services specifically for their age group via the Child and Adolescent Mental Health Services (CAMHS), while parents access Adult Mental Health Services, and Social Services respond to 'child in need' or 'child at risk' presentations. In CAMHS, generally, assessment and interventions are focused on the child or young person in the context of their home life and family structure. Likewise, therapeutic work is oriented towards the needs of the child or young person. If a parent's mental health issues become evident, they are usually signposted towards an appropriate adult-focused service where assessment and/or treatment can be made available. It would be unusual for the CAMHS service to attempt to 'treat' the parent at the same time as the child or young person.

Outside the UK, other approaches have been found. Handley *et al.* (2001), in their Australian study looking at the needs of children with a parent or carers with mental health issues, reported that mental health services were designed for the adults only and that there was a gap in provision, which meant that the needs of this vulnerable group, which they called 'the invisible children', were left unmet. Maybery and Reupert (2009) also highlighted the challenge of creating mental health services that are family-focused, with effective organisational structures and adequately trained staff who could meet the needs of parents and their children in families where parents had been affected by mental health issues.

There are some areas of work that involve whole families, such as systemic family therapy approaches, or family work in psychosis, but routine mental health services for either adults or children do not customarily offer a family-centred approach to assessment and intervention for both adults and children in families affected by mental health issues. Even in some of these family work approaches, such as behavioural family intervention for psychosis (see Chapter 3), children are often excluded from the therapeutic process.

Aims and learning outcomes

The aim of this chapter is to explore the challenges facing families where one or both parents experience mental health issues, and how these challenges may present in caring for their children's needs. Having completed the chapter, the reader will:

- Have an understanding of the issues facing children when their parents experience mental health issues
- Have an overview of some helpful approaches for families living with this situation
- Gain an ability to consider the mental health needs of the whole family in an integrated way.

Why is it important to specifically consider the mental health issues of parents?

There are two perspectives that need to be considered when thinking about the experiences of families in which there are parents with mental health issues: firstly the needs of the children living within that family; and secondly the needs of the parents who are balancing the role of parenting with the other stressors they are dealing with.

The needs of children within the family

There is evidence suggesting that children of parents with mental health issues (COPMI) are at increased risk of experiencing mental health issues themselves – certainly more so than the general population (Jessop & DeBondt 2012, Rutter 1989). Research shows that serious parental mental illness is associated with increased risk of adverse outcomes in children. In a systematic review of the available evidence, it was found that the short-term outcomes for these children included poorer mental and physical health as well as increased risk of a range of behavioural, social and educational difficulties. Such difficulties occurring at developmentally significant times are likely to have long-term consequences. The review also found that such long-term outcomes could sometimes extend into adulthood. These outcomes included social or occupational dysfunction, lower self-esteem, increased psychiatric morbidity and alcohol or substance misuse (Bee *et al.* 2014).

One possible reason for this phenomenon is that a parent with mental health issues might sometimes be less able to offer consistent emotional support for their child, or (as a consequence of their own lability of mood or experience of troublesome symptoms) may live in a social situation that makes them vulnerable to emotional, financial and social family burden (Devlin & O'Brien, 1999). There appears to be evidence of intergenerational transferability of mental health issues (Solantaus *et al.* 2010). Whether this is because of physiological or sociological reasons is not yet clear, but we do know that patterns of mental health issues can transcend the generations.

In their study of children of parents with mental health issues, Handley *et al.* (2001) found that children experienced distinct areas of need. Children had difficulty understanding the nature of their parents' mental illness, what it was, what the symptoms were, and what was happening to their parent. In some cases, children were worrying excessively about their parent and at other times they were trying to provide care for them.

This study also found that some children generally had difficulty talking about their parents' mental health issues so they did not talk about them at all. Other children were embarrassed about their parents' mental health issues and this affected their ability to talk about them. Handley *et al.*'s work suggests some useful interventions that any health or social care professional might include in their approach to working with a family with parents who are affected by mental health issues. Helping the parents and children gain a shared understanding of the nature of the parent's health issue, using language and materials suited to the developmental age of the child(ren) might be very helpful to the whole family because it informs the children, and helps empower the parents to have those conversations with them.

The experiences of the parents

One view is that parents with mental health issues themselves are experiencing significant amounts of stress related to their role as parents (Shor *et al.* 2015) and that this area of need goes unnoticed by healthcare professionals. However, a study investigating the experiences of parents with mental illness in the UK and Finland found that they experienced some aspects of parenting as stressful and others as helpful. They acknowledged that their mental health issues could be potentially disruptive to their family life but also reported that parenting gave them a sense of focus, and the responsibility associated with the parenting role was helpful to them (Jones *et al.* 2016). In other words, a mixed picture is emerging.

Occasionally, children who present to CAMHS live with parents who themselves have mental health issues and would like to access their own mental health assessment and/or treatment. In these situations, the CAMHS professional may refer the parent to an appropriate service (either a GP or a mental health professional). However, this referral does not allow for a consideration of the wider family-centred issues, such as how the needs of the parent and child are connected, how to organise appointments around childcare or school timings, and how to integrate the two sources of care provision. Similarly, if parents are being cared for in inpatient mental health facilities, there may be processes for arranging visits to the parents by their children, and these might be supervised where it is thought necessary. However these visits could also be seen as opportunities to use this time therapeutically, for practitioners to facilitate discussions and support between the parent and their children.

Intervention models for families where parental mental health is an issue

Child-focused interventions

The following section highlights a small number of standardised packages or individual interventions that might be useful in reducing distress in children whose parents experience mental health issues.

Solantaus *et al.* (2010) investigated two interventions designed to be preventative for children in families where one of the parents had a mood disorder. The 'Family Talk Interventions' and 'Let's Talk About Children' are both multi-session programmes. The Family Talk Intervention is a six-session package that enables parents to explore how to talk to their children about their symptoms of depression. In studying these two packages, Solantaus *et al.* found that they were helpful and clinically effective in 'decreasing children's emotional symptoms, anxiety, and marginally hyperactivity and in improving children's prosocial behaviour'. Parents were also given a self-help guide. There is a self-help guide available from MIND called *How to cope as a parent with a mental health problem* (MIND 2013). These programmes were designed to enhance communication in families where mood disorders were problematic, and also to increase resilience in children by developing their social connections and building on their strengths.

A Dutch study found that support groups for 8- to 12-year-olds whose parents had mental health issues were effective in improving cognition, social support and social acceptance (van Santvoort *et al.* 2014). In the structured package they used role-play so that children could rehearse how they might respond to a range of potentially uncomfortable social situations related to their parents' mental health. They also watched videotaped material produced by other children in similar situations, describing their experiences. However, the researchers did not note any improvement in the child-parent interaction as a result of the support groups and, perhaps because the intervention was offered too late, there was no improvement generally in the children's emotional or behavioural problems. It may be that support groups are indicated for some children, but that the needs of children with parents who have mental health issues need to be determined individually.

Parent-focused interventions

Shor *et al.* (2015) investigated the usefulness of a supportive group for parents who were accessing outpatient mental health services. The facilitated group work aimed to offer psycho-educational interventions to promote group members' understanding of how their mental health issues impacted on their parenting roles, to offer a space for peer support to develop, and to explore ways of overcoming any barriers to accessing relevant services.

Shor *et al.*'s study also looked at how parents maintain relationships with their children during periods when their children were not living with them and how hard that was for them, highlighting how it could lead to insecurity and lack of self-confidence as parents. The reported benefits of discussing this in a peer group included a sharing of ideas on how to address this, and a sharing of activities that others had found successful. Emotional support was another positive effect of this group work approach. As the group consisted of parents with mental health issues, all shared some common experiences and either expressed concern about living away from their children or fear that their children would be removed. Open discussion about these concerns was found to be cathartic. Participants in the group were encouraged by their peers in their attempts to continue trying to connect with their children. They also found it helpful to explore ways of talking to their children about mental health issues they were experiencing as well as getting advice on how to do that differently, and in an age-appropriate way.

A model for consultation for healthcare practitioners working in adult mental health services with parents has been developed in Queensland, Australia. The consultation is offered by a small team from the child mental health service, to assist the mental health practitioners in adult metal health services in developing a comprehensive family assessment, providing brief family-focused interventions and, where relevant, assisting in referral to other services (Jessop & De Bondt 2012). Through this process, some adolescents were identified for referral to a specific intervention to increase their coping skills, and a COPMI champion was identified in the adult mental health services to take the lead. This model could be adopted elsewhere, where relationships between adult mental health services and CAMHS exist.

Bee *et al.* (2014) conducted an evidence synthesis to look at the clinical effectiveness, cost effectiveness and acceptability of community-based interventions aimed at improving the quality of life for children of parents with serious mental illness. They categorised their findings into four groups as follows: psychotherapy, psycho-education, psychosocial and complex interventions. This review had two arms: one focused around research specifically addressing families where a defined serious mental illness had been diagnosed (such as schizophrenia, schizo-affective disorder, bipolar affective disorder, puerperal psychosis, borderline personality disorder); and the other addressing families where members had severe unipolar or post-natal depression. It should be noted that of the 29 trials included in the review, only six included the outcomes of fathers or partners. Nor did the review look at evidence for interventions for anxiety or mild to moderate mental health issues, or addiction issues or eating disorders.

However, this 2014 review did identify that most of the interventions were focused on the health of the parent with serious mental health issues, or on improving symptoms or symptom management. In addition, the interventions were generally delivered at an individual level, typically using cognitive behavioural therapy. Only 40% of the studies included in the review specifically looked at interventions designed to enhance parenting or family function, and just 9 of the 43 interventions reported were directly delivered to children.

In the summary of this useful review, there is a suggestion that, despite the lack of evidence about fathers, mild to moderate mental health issues and child- or parent-focused interventions, there is some hope that whole family assessments can be conducted in community settings and that adult mental health services will be accessible to parents affected by mental health. Group-based interventions aimed at challenging stigma appear to be useful. Importantly, the report suggests that there should be no assumptions about effectiveness related to whether or not the child is resident with the parent affected by mental health.

Family-focused interventions

There is a third sector organisation, called Our Time (2019), which specifically supports young people affected by parental mental illness. Within its range of services, there are resources for both parents and children, for professionals, support groups and information. The *Think child, think parent, think family report* (Social Care Institute for Excellence 2009) recommended a number of pragmatic ways of working with the whole family, where parental mental illness is an issue. Taking a strengths-based approach with families is recommended as an option that allows a reframing of the home situation, acknowledging the strengths within the family and enabling the family to draw on these to manage difficulties or emerging problems. The use of a family conference is suggested as a method of encouraging solution finding within a family, all members contributing to a process of discussion and sharing ideas on how to overcome a presenting difficulty.

Ways forward

Thinking about community services

Jessop and De Bondt (2012) suggest some reasons why there is not yet an expansive service that meets the needs of families where a parent is experiencing mental health issues. One of the reasons postulated is that the practitioners are worried they lack the skills needed to work with both adults and children. In Australia, in response to this perceived training need, a web-based training package 'The Keeping Families and Children in Mind: COPMI Mental Health Worker Education Resource' was developed by the Australian Infant, Child, Adolescent and Family Mental Health Association.

One model that might have wide utility is the consultation approach used in Brisbane (discussed above). This has a number of component parts: training, consultation between child mental health and adult mental health services, intervention to enhance coping skills for children, and establishing COPMI champions in adult mental health services. Ideally all aspects would be adopted, but the inclusion of any of the component parts might be helpful for families where parents experience mental health issues.

Inpatient services

Thus far, this discussion has focused on families where the parent is receiving care as an outpatient, whether or not the child is currently living in the same home. However, there is another context that needs consideration. When a parent is admitted to an inpatient facility, this can have a profound effect on their child. The circumstances surrounding the admission might need to be explained to the child, as might the reason for a prolonged or hasty admission into hospital. This is potentially a frightening experience for the child – more so if they need to live with other caregivers, such as family or foster carers for a time.

In this situation, it may be helpful to have a selection of age-appropriate information sources (such as leaflets, DVDs and online resources) readily available for parents to give their children, a dedicated child-friendly visiting area and healthcare practitioners who are skilled in facilitating contact between patients who are parents and their children. Competence in talking to children and young people using age-appropriate language and media, as well as knowledge of simple strategies for reducing anxiety and distress, would be a good start.

Practitioner skills

Roth, Calder and Pilling (2013) have developed a framework that maps the competencies required for professionals working with children and young people at various levels of engagement. This framework was designed with children's mental health provision in mind, but it could be useful for all practitioners working in the field of mental health who are likely to encounter families where children are present. It might be used initially by services to benchmark what they believe a foundation level of competencies might be, and then to identify key individuals within that service to develop enhanced competencies through bespoke training, education or supervision packages.

The following are suggestions that might be included in our usual practice to move towards a service that can better meet the needs of a family affected by parental mental health issues.

If mental health services for adults were considered within the context of mental health promotion for their children, then family-centred work that promoted resilience and coping strategy enhancement might benefit the whole family. There is an emerging body of work promoting strategies to enhance the emotional resilience of children and young people. One definition of emotional resilience is the ability of children and young people to cope with the stressors of life, both expected and unexpected. A child living with a parent affected by mental health issues might be expected to experience stress more frequently, and thus any increase in their ability to cope with stress would be helpful for them. Enhancing resilience strategies typically include: helping children build good relationships with others, including adults and peers; helping children to develop their emotional intelligence, and identify, express and manage their emotions; and encouraging children to build their confidence by taking on personal challenges. The Beyond Blue Support Service offers a wide range of resilience resources on its website (Beyond Blue 2019).

Mental health services should be modified to accommodate family-focused interventions either for individual families or for groups of families (Devlin & O'Brien 1999), including elements of peer support, improving family functioning and strategies to reduce social isolation.

Illustrative case study

Mary has three school-aged children: Thomas is 12, Luke is 10 and Josh is 8. Mary is currently receiving care from a secondary mental health service for bipolar affective disorder. She has lived with this condition since the birth of her youngest son, and she goes through long periods of low mood characterised by difficulty in socialising and leaving the house. This is interspersed by periods when she is 'her usual self', when she can engage in active parenting, being busy at home and helping younger children at school with the supported reading scheme. Mary's husband John works full-time as a contractor, and often works late into the evening and occasional weekends.

Luke was referred and assessed by the local CAMHS, where he was found to be displaying symptoms suggestive of anxiety. Mary was also concerned about her oldest son Thomas. Although the youngest son Josh was quiet throughout the CAMHS consultation, Mary did not raise any concerns about him. Both older boys thought Josh was not himself – sullen and sad, did not join in playing with them at home and hid himself in his bedroom for long periods.

In this family, rather than assess and intervene with the children separately from the mother, it would seem useful to consider the whole family as a unit. In order to successfully achieve this, the CAMHS and adult community mental health team met with the family for a one-off consultation. This allowed them to have a conversation about the needs of everyone in the family and how services might work together to support them. The interventions offered included psycho-education about both the presentations of the children and of Mary, some shared family support mechanisms or resilience building, and an opportunity to think with Mary and John how they could continue to effectively parent the children – drawing on their resources outside the immediate family unit (such as support from grandparents).

Suggested reflection and further activities

If working with people with mental health issues, routinely ask if they are parents, determining the details of age, location and current care provision for their children. Fathers are forgotten more often than mothers (Jones *et al.* 2016) so you should routinely ask men who access mental health services if they are parents too and explore with them their needs relating to parenting their children.

In your working context, consider how you might address the needs of these parents and their children. Ideas that might be helpful for improving services for parents and their children affected by mental health issues include: creating a clear pathway for liaison with other agencies (including the adult/CAMHS mental health interface); offering information about health issues and treatments that covers a breadth of age and reading levels, and is therefore appropriate for parents to access with their children; and providing specific group support for parents, children or both.

To develop services that are more family-focused and can better respond to the needs of parents affected by mental health issues, invite people who have become expert through their own experiences to consult and advise on service development.

- How might you enhance your skills and knowledge to better prepare you to work with these families?
- How confident are you in your understanding of child development?
- How might it be possible to collaborate with a colleague from a complementary area of clinical practice?

Conclusion

In this chapter the needs of parents with mental health issues have been considered, and we have discussed approaches to working solely with parents, solely with children, and with the whole family. Many adults who access mental health services are parents. We need to ask about parenting-related issues when we assess people's needs and ensure that we include family-focused approaches in our intervention plans and support services. Parents with mental health issues often avoid disclosure for fear that they will be considered unable to parent their children safely and effectively. Fathers' parenting roles are often forgotten. There is clearly an opportunity for different agencies and services to work together to better meet the needs of families affected by mental health issues.

Recommended reading

MIND (2013). *How to cope as a parent with a mental health problem.* https://www.mind.org.uk/media/447394/how-to-cope-as-a-parent-with-a-mental-health-problem-2013.pdf (last accessed 7.8.2019). This publication offers a good foundation for signposting to families.

Roth, A.D., Calder, F. & Pilling, S. (2013). *A competence framework for Child and Adolescent Mental Health Services.* https://www.ucl.ac.uk/clinical-psychology//CORE/child-adolescent-competences/CAMHS%20Competences%20Framework_V1%20(2).pdf The competency framework is useful for self-development as well as service development, as it enables practitioners to identify the skill set currently available and what competencies it would be useful to develop to meet the needs of children and young people at various stages.

References

Bee, P., Bower, P., Byford, S., Churchill, R., Calam, R., Stallard, P., Pryjmachuk, S., Berzins, K., Cary, M., Wan, M. & Abel, K. (2014). The clinical effectiveness, cost-effectiveness and acceptability of community-based interventions aimed at improving or maintaining quality of life in children of parents with serious mental illness: a systematic review. *National Institute for Health Research.* DOI: 10.3310/hta18080

Beyond Blue (2019). https://healthyfamilies.beyondblue.org.au/healthy-homes/building-resilience (last accessed 30.9.2019).

Boursnell, M. (2014). Assessing the capacity of parents with mental illness: parents with mental illness and risk. *International Social Work.* **57**, 92–108.

Devlin, J.M. & O'Brien, L.M. (1999). Children of parents with mental illness: An overview from a nursing perspective. *Australian and New Zealand Journal of Mental Health Nursing.* **8**, 19–29.

Handley, C., Farrell, G.A., Josephs, A., Hanke, A. & Hazelton, M. (2001). The Tasmanian children's project: the needs of children with a parent/carer with a mental illness. *Australian and New Zealand Journal of Mental Health Nursing.* **10**, 221–28.

Jessop, M.E. & De Bondt, N. (2012). A consultation service for Adult Mental Health Service clients who are parents and their families. *Advances in Mental Health.* **10** (2), 149–56.

Jones, M., Pietila, I., Joronen, K., Simpson, W., Gray, S. & Kaunonen, M. (2016). Parents with mental illness – a qualitative study of identities and experiences with support services. *Journal of Psychiatric and Mental Health Nursing.* **23**, 471–78.

Maybery, D. & Reupert, A. (2009). Parental mental illness: a review of barriers and issues for working with families and children. *Journal of Psychiatric and Mental Health Nursing.* **156**, 784–91.

MIND (2013). *How to cope as a parent with a mental health problem.* https://www.mind.org.uk/media/447394/how-to-cope-as-a-parent-with-a-mental-health-problem-2013.pdf (last accessed 7.8.2019).

Our Time (2019). https://OurTime.org.uk (last accessed 30.9.2019).

Roth, A.D., Calder, F. & Pilling, S. (2013). *A competence framework for Child and Adolescent Mental Health Services.* https://www.ucl.ac.uk/clinical-psychology//CORE/child-adolescent-competences/CAMHS%20Competences%20Framework_V1%20(2).pdf (last accessed 7.8.2019).

Royal College of Psychiatrists (2014). *Parental Mental Illness: The impact on children and adolescents; Information for parents, carers and anyone who works with young people.* London: Royal College of Psychiatrists.

Rutter, M. (1989). 'Psychiatric Disorder in parents as a risk factor for children.' In: V. Anthon, N.B. Enzer, I. Phillips, D. Shaffer & M.M. Silverman (eds). *Prevention of Mental Disorders, Alcohol and Other Drug Use in Children and Adolescents, OSAP Prevention Monograph – 2*. Rockville, Maryland: Office for Substance Abuse Prevention.

Shor, R., Kalivatz, Z., Amir, Y., Aldor, R. & Lipot, M. (2015). Therapeutic factors in a group for parents with mental illness. *Community Mental Health Journal.* **51**, 79–84.

Social Care Institute for Excellence (SCIE) (2009). *Think Child, Think Parent, Think Family: A Guide to Parental Mental Health and Child Welfare.* London: SCIE.

Solantaus, T., Paavonen, E.J., Toikka, S., & Punamäki, R. (2010). Preventive interventions in families with parental depression: children's psychosocial symptoms and prosocial behaviour. *European Child and Adolescent Psychiatry.* **19**, 883–92.

van Santvoort, F., Hosman, C.M.H., van Doesum, K.T.M., & Janssens, J.M.A.M. (2014). Effectiveness of preventive support groups for children of mentally ill or addicted parents: a randomized controlled trial. *European Child and Adolescent Psychiatry.* **23**, 473–84.

Chapter 5

Understanding moment-by-moment interactions in families: assessment and treatment utilising a domains framework

S. Riley, J. Hill, H. Lee and P. Tranter

Introduction

The study of human interaction has always been at the heart of sociological endeavour, especially from the perspective of community life. The value of understanding interactional processes in the family as a means of assessing and treating the mental health needs of children and young people is well recognised (AFT 2016, Stratton 2016). The question of how to utilise family interaction and processes continues to be debated, especially from an epistemological and ethical perspective and within a therapeutic and practice delivery context.

In this chapter we aim to explore family interactional processes in the form of a conceptual framework, and we will also look at the practical applications of this framework. We consider the domains framework as a resource which enhances the mental health practitioner's knowledge, and their ability to carry out assessments and put theory into practice when working with families. The domains framework provides practitioners with a way of understanding a family's moment-by-moment interactions. Understanding and influencing interaction in family life can contribute to improving patterns of interaction, which may subsequently enhance the quality of relationships. We believe that improving the quality of moment-by-moment interaction can help in the management of emotional distress and arguments; increase warmth and understanding of when and how to give comfort; decrease confusion; and increase mutual problem-solving and ability to reflect.

Aims and learning outcomes

Having completed this chapter, the reader will have:
- An understanding of the fundamental concepts of social domains

- An ability to identify domains and judge whether they are clear or unclear, and matched or mismatched
- A knowledge of how to aid observation and reporting of family interaction.

Domains framework

The aim of this chapter is to provide an approach to listening to, and observing, what happens between parents and children, and between mental health professionals, parents and young people. It introduces a framework for doing this that draws on developmental research into parent–child interactions and adds ideas on how these fit together. Bringing the observations and the theory together can lead to new understanding that can be shared with parents and young people, which in turn generates ideas for alternative solutions in therapeutic and wider clinical work.

To do this we make use of the 'Social Domains Framework' (Hill, Fonagy, Safier & Sargent 2003; Hill, Wren, Alderton *et al.* 2014) which proposes that social interactions of all kinds, and between all people, can take place quickly and satisfactorily when participants have a shared set of rules for interpreting other people's behaviours, and especially emotional states, and for responding to them. These are referred to as social domains, which Bugental (2000) elegantly characterised as 'algorithms of social life'. Much of this chapter focuses on domains of interaction between parents and children; we also review how the domains approach can be applied to interactions between clinicians and parents, and between children and parents/carers. In general, a domains analysis will be particularly relevant when interactions between participants have become intense or sustained, which is obviously the case in families, but also sometimes for practitioners, especially in Child and Adolescent Mental Health Services (CAMHS) inpatient settings.

Basic assumptions

- Everything that people say and do in family life carries information about the type of interaction they are engaged in (Hill *et al.* 2014).
- One part of the family cannot be understood in isolation from the rest of the system (Epstein, Bishop & Levin 1978).
- Transactional patterns in family systems are involved in shaping the behaviour of family members (Epstein *et al.* 1978).
- Communication which is unclear and/or indirect can contribute to interpersonal problems (Will & Wrate 1985), resulting in misunderstandings, irresolvable arguments or distress (Hill *et al.* 2014).
- Work with children's and young people's mental health often requires parents/carers to be co-therapists.

Interactional rules are obvious in games with explicit rules, such as football or Monopoly, but less obvious in the majority of social interactions, which are often implicit, and usually more fluid and complex. Family interactions (which include verbal and non-verbal communication) are often fluid, and at the same time occur without awareness of the underlying rules. This does not matter when there is harmony and understanding and problems are solved effectively. However, in families where interactions are confusing, conflicted or distressing, or problems remain unsolved, identifying and clarifying the underlying rules (domains) can provide a basis for finding new solutions. The same is true of interactions between professionals, parents and young people, which can be particularly demanding when a young person has a mental health problem. The analysis can be applied to all clinicians, but in this chapter we will focus on nursing.

An illustrative example

Here is an example of a typical family interaction, of a mother greeting her daughter when she comes in from school:

Mother: Hi, what kind of a day have you had?

Within a domains framework, this greeting by a parent belongs in a social domain. Even on the basis of this short utterance, we can describe the most likely domain, and the alternatives, and what it is about the communication that would push us one way or another in our understanding of what is being said and how to respond. We can also describe the domain a young person (YP) might experience this to be in. Once we have established the meaning of what has been communicated, we are in a better position to understand how a greeting like this may lead to a distressing argument, with negative consequences for family relationships and mental health.

For example:

Mother says that she asked her daughter how her day was.

Within the domains framework, this general characterisation may imply a domain, but it is not specific enough to determine which one. Only once we know the words the mother used to enquire, and how she spoke, are we in a position to start to explore the domains.

In this interaction, the parent's intention may be:

Mother tried to find out how her day was.

At this point, the communication provides little indication of the domain and needs further understanding.

What are the domains?

According to the domains framework, interactions between parents and their YP take place in four domains – **Safety, Attachment, Discipline/Expectation** and

Exploratory. Apart from Safety, the dynamics of these domains have been extensively researched (Hill *et al.* 2014).

In **Safety** parents do their best to ensure that their child does not come to harm, and in doing this they take direct action or prescribe what should happen, insisting with authority, and if necessary, against the wishes or feelings of the young person, and making clear to the young person why they are acting in this way. Imagine a young child and their parent are out on a bike ride and they come across a steep hill and the child immediately wants to ride their bike down a steep hill. The parent and child interaction when clearly in the safety domain might be something like:

> Parent: STOP, George. It's not safe – that hill is too steep to ride down.
> George: But I'll be OK.
> Parent: It's not safe, you could hurt yourself. We'll get off the bikes and walk down.
> George: OK.

Another example might involve a young adolescent who has just unwittingly opened a risky website. As in the example above, the parent has a responsibility to respond quickly to safeguard their young person, with a simple but clear instruction about safety:

> Parent: That website is not safe, close it down.
> Melanie: OK, I was only looking for a picture of an X-man.
> Parent: Yes, but the search has brought up dangerous websites. Close it down for now, we can search together safely later.

In **Attachment** the parent's role is to do their best to understand their child's distress, worries, fears or sadness. They respond to their child's emotions or behaviours at the young person's pace, following their feelings, and keeping the focus on the young person's (rather than their own) needs.

Imagine a child signals their distress (e.g. they are tearful or uncommonly quiet) following a falling-out with their friend or sibling.

[Parent communicates tentatively, enquiring and listening for understanding]

> Mary: (Tearfully) Mum.
> Mother: (Stopping to illustrate a focusing and willingness to listen and in a tender voice) What is the matter? Come and sit down.
> Mary: (Still tearful) Jack shouted at me for using his bike and said he hates me.
> Mother: I see you're upset. (Mum gives Mary a hug)
> Mary: He's never going to speak to me again.
> Mother: Shall we see if we can sort this out? Or are you still too upset?
> Mary: OK. (Mum stays with Mary's emotions as long as needed)

Now consider a 15-year-old young person returning from being out with friends. She signals her distress/attachment/need by throwing her bag down abruptly.

    Dad: That's not like you. What's the matter, El?

    Ellie: Doesn't matter.

    Dad: What's up? Can I help or do you need some space?
    (Said in concerned and kind tone)

    Ellie: Need some space.

    Dad: OK, shall I make a brew and bring it through?

    Ellie: OK.

    Some time later...

    Dad: Here you are, El. Are you ready to talk?

    Ellie: Yeah, Katy and Hannah were ignoring me on the bus – texting each other.

    Dad: That's not nice, you must have felt left out.

    Ellie: Yeah, it's just mean and I wouldn't do it to them.

    Dad: Do you know why they were behaving that way? Looks like they have really upset you.

    Ellie: I feel really sad, I thought they were good friends.

    Dad: Feeling sad is not very nice... Shall we do something together... Shall we make tea? Or do you need more time to work out how you feel?

    Ellie: Yeah, I'll come and help you in a minute.

    Dad: Are you sure you don't want me to stay?

    Ellie: I'll be OK, thanks. I'm starting to feel better.

A key feature of the interaction within the Attachment Domain is that the parent stays with the young person until the young person's distress goes, whilst also using space and appropriate timing. Parental responses would be adjusted depending on the young person's developmental age.

In **Discipline/Expectation** parents teach their child which behaviours are acceptable and unacceptable, and encourage them to tackle challenges, insisting with authority (and, if necessary, against the wishes or feelings of the young person) and making clear to the young person why they are acting in this way. Communication in the Expectation Domain is influenced by the developmental processes that normally occur during maturation, with parents modifying levels of expectation in accordance with the maturity of the young person.

Consider a young child who is in the throes of pouring a carton of milk over the cat and the front room carpet.

Mother: Charlie, STOP...that is naughty.

Charlie continues with his actions.

Mother: Stop that. You will have to go to your room if you continue.

Charlie stops.

Mother: Right, let's get a towel and tidy up.

Now consider a conversation with an older adolescent.

Kate: I'm off out now.

Mum: I want you home for 9pm.

Kate: Can I stay out until 9.30? Everybody else does.

Mum: No, be home at 9 and no later. You've got school in the morning.

In **Exploratory** parents and children share together whatever is important or a source of pleasure to them: experiences, plans, music, jokes, watching TV or thoughts. They talk about what they think and listen to each other's ideas, and in doing this they contribute equally, showing interest, without parents insisting when a young person does not want to share. Fundamentally this is moment-by-moment interaction which does not call for any action to be taken by anyone.

The domains framework allows for developmental changes, as children's behaviours and parents' responses change as children get older. At some point during adolescence they change a lot because parents take less responsibility for their young people's safety, and for teaching them what are acceptable behaviours, but the principles remain the same. The process of negotiation occurs much more often with older adolescents.

From moment to moment, parents make choices based on their children's behaviours, and on their judgements about those behaviours, regarding the domain in which they respond. Family life is often very fast-moving and decisions (especially those regarding a child's safety or their aggressive or disruptive outbursts) sometimes have to be made quickly. Problems can occur when cues are unclear (low domain clarity) such as distress following separation (attachment), or opposition when asked to tidy up (discipline). The signals may be brief or difficult for a parent to spot. Furthermore, from the child's perspective, the parent's response may not make the domain clear, so the rules for solving problems, dealing with emotions and for understanding each other may then also not be clear. The clarity is affected by the extent to which each of the distinctive features of the domain is present. When we talk to parents or families about the domains, we often illustrate this using the grid shown in Table 5.1 below.

Table 5.1: The domains framework

Domains – Clear channels			
Exploratory	Safety	Attachment	Expectation
Is there something to solve?			
NO	YES	YES	YES
Who takes responsibility?			
SHARED	PARENT	PARENT	PARENT
Whose pace do you go at?			
CHILD	PARENT	CHILD	PARENT
Do you respond to your child's wishes and emotions?			
YES	NO	YES	NO
Do you emphasise the difference in hierarchy between child and parent?			
NO	YES	YES	YES
How do you sound?			
INTERESTED	DEFINITE	TENDER	DETERMINED
How do you look?			
INTERESTED	DEFINITE	TENDER	DETERMINED
How much time do you want to spend in it?			
AS MUCH AS POSSIBLE	AS LITTLE AS POSSIBLE	AS MUCH AS NEEDED	AS LITTLE AS POSSIBLE

Illustrative examples highlighting different domain interactions

Example 1 (relatively straightforward):
A young person comes home from school and says, 'Helena said something very unfair to me, it really upset me.' This is almost certainly a clear Attachment bid, looking for some sympathy or even comfort from a parent. (We say 'almost certainly' because the bid will be clear if the young person conveys sadness or upset, but less clear if they sound angry.)

Example 2 (relatively straightforward):
A young person comes home from school and says, 'There's a party on Saturday and I am going.' Usually this type of statement calls for a Discipline/Expectation response from a parent indicating whether or not that is acceptable; or, if the parent is concerned about safety issues, such as drugs or violence, a Safety response.

Example 3 (complex):
A young person comes home from school and says nothing. The parent says 'how was school?' If the parent says this lightly, sounding interested, it is clearly Exploratory. If the parent sounds angry or stern, it will be unclear whether it is Exploratory or Discipline/

Expectation. The young person says 'OK' in a grumpy tone, without looking at the parent. This is not a clear bid for a domain. It could reflect unhappiness (indicating Attachment); or it could reflect Discipline/Expectation because it is rude; or it could be what the young person says when they have self-harmed, in which case it is a cue for Safety; or it is an invitation for an Exploratory conversation.

The parent will probably be uncertain how to proceed, because the young person's signal is not clear, so they may say something like, 'What do you mean "OK"?' Even though the parent is feeling angry at being spoken to that way, or worried about what it means, if they say it lightly and with interest and without insistence this could be a clear Exploratory response. If the parent's question sounds somewhat impatient, or critical, or worried, the domain will be unclear to the young person. When the domain is unclear, it can lead to misunderstandings, anger or upset, because the parent and the young person are interpreting things differently or making different assumptions. The parent may be trying to show they are interested (Exploratory), but the young person hears criticism and interprets it as Discipline/Expectation. Then the parent feels that their attempts to help are being rejected, and the young person feels/thinks the parent does not understand. These are the kinds of difficult situations that can be helped by an understanding of domains.

The main point is that when the domain is clear, parent and young person know where they are with each other. In Attachment and Exploratory, a clear domain lays the foundation for understanding, comfort or sharing; and in Safety and Discipline/Expectation, a clear domain ensures that the young person knows the parent's stance and the reasons for it, even though they might not agree. If the domain is unclear, there can be confusion, and emotions can run high. For example, if a parent responds to a child's distress by saying something like, 'don't cry, there is no need for those tears', they may be aiming to comfort them. But if the parent sounds stern or angry, the child may hear something that sounds more like a Discipline instruction. Then the child does not know whether they are being comforted or told off. When the domain is unclear, it can therefore become much harder for the parent and young person to understand each other, and to resolve emotional upset.

This is also likely to be the case when the parent and young person are in different domains (which we refer to as a 'domain mismatch'). So, for example, if a child is crying because they are worried or frightened and the parent thinks they are doing it to get their own way, and gets angry with the child, parent and child are not in the same domain, and there is a domain mismatch. Then the child feels even more upset because the parent does not understand, and is not offering them comfort; and the parent gets more upset because the child seems to be stubborn and self-willed.

More on the Exploratory domain

In the Exploratory domain, parents and children enjoy being together, playing, joking, teasing, going on outings, or just talking about their day or what film they have seen. The Exploratory domain can also be quite serious – for example, if parents and children are talking over something important, or trying to sort out a misunderstanding. However, when they are in the Exploratory domain, parents and children are not usually distressed or angry. In contrast to the other domains, in which the parent makes hierarchy clear, in the Exploratory domain the parent and child are more like equals. For example, the parent remembers something that happened during the day, then the child adds something else; or the child talks about something they like doing and the parent adds something else.

In the Exploratory domain the parent does not try to create certainty; in fact they do the opposite. The Exploratory domain works best when the parent does not try to impose control, but makes the child feel that at least two people are needed to keep things going. So, when parents relate through an Exploratory conversation, they should talk in a way that does not sound stern and makes it easy for the child to respond. We talk about family members embracing uncertainty when they are in the Exploratory domain. Unlike the other domains (which are often best kept as short as possible), the longer family members remain Exploratory, the more they enjoy being together and the better they come to understand each other.

There are two big potential gains when a parent responds to a young person in the Exploratory domain. First, because the parent is not stern or annoyed (as in the Discipline domain), the young person does not need to work out how to regulate their own emotions, and so is likely to be able to think things out. Second, Exploratory exchanges can add information, which usually does not happen in the domains of Safety, Attachment or Discipline. This gives the parent better guidance on what to do. So often, especially with adolescents, it can be helpful to respond where possible in the Exploratory domain. Even when the young person may appear to be oppositional or not meeting expectations, further information may clarify whether or not this is really the case.

Imagine a young person rings up late in the evening from town, saying they cannot get home. Instinctively the parent, assuming that they will have to go and get them and feeling they should be able to manage this at their age, responds in Discipline/Expectation, angrily saying something like 'it's not that late, find a bus'. There then follows an argument. If the parent responds with enquiries, in Exploratory mode, embracing uncertainty (asking where the young person is exactly, who with, asking if they have seen buses, found a timetable, etc.), the parent has a much stronger base from which either to advise in Exploratory or take action in Discipline/Expectation domain.

Sometimes it is in these sorts of conversations that something really important to guide the domain comes up. For instance, perhaps the young person has just had an argument with a friend or spent all their money. When the parent starts in the Exploratory domain, they support the young person in thinking things through without having to worry about how to respond to an angry parent and they also get more information to guide them on how to solve things.

More on domain clarity

Family life would be straightforward if parents and young people displayed notices or held up flags at all times to indicate which domain they were in, or trying to be in. In reality, the signals are often less than clear, and the action is fast-moving, so tracking domains can be difficult. Domains are indicated by a combination of what family members say and do. When words and actions all indicate one domain, people know where they are; when they indicate different domains, it becomes harder.

Take the very simple example of the young person coming in from school and the parent saying, 'Hi, how was school today?' That sounds like a clear Exploratory enquiry from a parent interested in what their child has been doing. But try varying the way it might be said – for example, placing the emphasis on 'today' seems to pick out today compared to yesterday. It might then sound like 'did you get in trouble today, like you did yesterday?' in which case is the domain Exploratory or Discipline? Suppose the young person says 'fine' but with their head down and sounding negative. It is then unclear whether they are irritated, angry or upset. The parent has very little to go on in responding, and we can imagine a wide range of things a parent might say, and then work out what domain they would each convey. This kind of exercise can be illuminating – trying out several ways in which a parent might respond. Suppose, for example, a parent said, 'is that it?' If spoken lightly and tentatively, that could keep the Exploratory domain clear; but spoken with irritation, or insistently, it could also sound like Discipline/Expectation, so the domain would not be clear.

More generally, when the features of the domain line up together, it is clear; and when they don't, it can be unclear. Domains can also be difficult to interpret in other forms of communication, such as text messages, where there is no non-verbal communication to interpret and the use of emojis, nicknames and kisses at the end of sentences can confuse things further.

Why try to understand family domains?

Most of the time we just get on with family life, and families move from one domain to another without thinking about it very much. However, experience tells us that it can sometimes be helpful to pause and try to work out how the domains are operating in the family. This is probably most truly the case where one or more family members are often getting angry or upset, or where there are disagreements that do not seem to come to a conclusion.

Thinking about domains can be very helpful if one of the family members has mental health problems. For example, depression is in some ways like sadness, which calls for the care and comfort of the Attachment domain. However, there are sometimes worries that the depression sufferer may harm themselves, and then the main issue is Safety. Equally, the depressed adolescent may need encouragement to do more things, in which case something more like the Discipline/Expectation domain is needed. Often family members find themselves trying to do more than one thing at a time, which is the normal response, but also runs the risk of creating 'low domain clarity' or 'domain mismatch', in which two domains are operating at the same time.

Below are two examples of tracking domains interaction in a family therapy session. These vignettes give the reader an opportunity to consider the moment-by-moment communication which illustrates the speed of conversations and how they can contribute to either problem-solving or disharmony, leading to relational difficulties. As previously mentioned, relationship difficulties are recognised as perpetuating factors influencing mental wellbeing.

One of the benefits of the domain framework is that it is transferable and pan-therapeutic (for example, it can also be used in CBT, Parenting, Family Work and other Psychosocial interventions). The framework has a practical use when young people come to the attention of Mental Health Services, particularly when they attend CAMHS. The authors have applied this framework in their clinical settings, working with young people, parents and families experiencing mental health problems. Specific work has been undertaken with young people who self-harm, and preliminary research in this area is currently being undertaken. The issues of low domain clarity and mismatch are frequently noted in children and young people with mental health difficulties and neurodevelopment needs. In this chapter we have chosen to focus on one specific presentation that commonly arises in CAMHS settings.

Domains functioning in relation to young people who self-harm

Rates of self-harm amongst young people have increased dramatically and dealing with this issue has become a common occurrence for front-line health care services and more specialist services. These young people often have rapidly changing and intense moods, and they may self-harm repeatedly. Such characteristics are likely to make interactions with their parents more difficult and distressing, and domains processes are consequently likely to be more difficult for parents and young people.

The challenge associated with rapidly changing and intense moods is that they can be difficult to read – the young person may look very different from how they feel inside. For example, a young person who is worried may look angry. The challenge with self-harm is that a parent could feel they need to respond in any of the domains, because it is a risk. The young person could be expressing distress or anger, or they could be attempting to communicate. Parents may inadvertently find they are trying to respond in several domains at the same time, leading to what we call low domain clarity. The challenge with feeling easily criticised is that something said to a young person in the Exploratory domain, such as an interested enquiry, may feel to the young person like a criticism, and so more like a Discipline/Expectation issue.

Things may also get confusing because parents, who are aware that their son or daughter is struggling with several difficulties, often try to help in more than one area of their life at the same time. For instance, consider a scenario in which a parent thinks their son or daughter could be putting themselves at risk. They may be wanting to help relieve their son or daughter's distress and ask them how they are feeling, intending to convey the Attachment domain. However, due to their own anxiety, they may inadvertently do it with the urgency of the Safety domain. The domain therefore becomes unclear and the young person feels something like 'my parent *seems* to be interested in how I feel, but *really* only wants to know if I am going to self-harm'. Quite possibly the parent's change of vocal pace or tone has occurred without them realising, so the young person feels angry at what they see as an intrusion, while the parent does not understand how this could have happened.

Illustrative case study

Sally is a sixteen-year-old with a history of chronic and severe self-harming behaviour. She returns from college having had some sad news about a friend who has been hospitalised. On getting home, Sally's mum greets her:

Dialogue	Track domain interaction
Mum: Hi, what kind of a day have you had?	*Exploratory, depending on tone and delivery*
Sally grunts and throws her school bag on the floor and storms upstairs.	*Low domain clarity*

Mum and Sally have an exchange as she storms upstairs to her room:

Mum: Hey, I only asked, young lady!!!	*Discipline*
Sally: Just shut up and leave me alone.	*Mum's hierarchy undermined*
Mum: I was just asking you what kind of day you have had.	*Low domain clarity*

Sally: Stop going on.	*Domain mismatch, young person in Discipline domain and Mum feels told off – hierarchy undermined*

Sometime later, asking through a closed door:

Mum: Do you want a cup of tea?	*Domains clear – Exploratory*
Sally: No just go away! You just don't get it, you don't care.	*Attachment bid – made difficult due to angry response*
Mum: I'll leave you alone, I'm just downstairs if you need me.	*Domain clear – attending to Attachment at Sally's pace*
Sally: Fine!!!!!'	*Low domain clarity*

Some time later, Sally remains silent in her room. Mum, becoming increasingly concerned, goes to check on her:

Mum: What are you up to in there?	*Low domain clarity – could be Discipline/Safety/Exploratory, depending on tone*
Sally: None of your business, just go away.	*Low domain clarity, Mum is hierarchically undermined*
Mum: I need to see if you are OK. I'm coming in.	*Safety*

Applying the domains framework in the context of CAMHS inpatient nursing

Applying the domains perspective to inpatient CAMHS nursing for children and adolescents with mental health problems can be very illuminating but it has to be done carefully. On the one hand, the domains are defined by the professional relationship between clinician and patient/client, but with the addition of the role of the practitioner in loco parentis. Whether or not the domains basis of the practitioner role is discussed and spelled out with parents (or even among staff), there is generally little doubt that practitioners have a Safety responsibility, and commonly have to adopt a Discipline/Expectation position. On the other hand, practitioners are not primarily Attachment figures and there is a limit to how far they can respond to attachment bids, and their role in relation to attachment processes is often ambiguous. One of the aims of nursing in inpatient services is to be Exploratory, in that they seek to collaborate with the child or young person to increase understanding, and so a significant aspect of the practitioner's therapeutic role centres around Exploratory interactions.

Take, for example, the question of whether an adolescent is 'engaged' with treatment. The domains-based approach first addresses which domains might be relevant for that patient. When a young person has psychotic experiences, it is often clear that staff take responsibility for the treatment, and the dynamics of the interaction mainly belong in the Safety domain. Contrast this with a young person who has engaged in self-harming behaviour or restricting their dietary intake, as in anorexia nervosa. To which domains does the term 'engagement' refer? Here enquiry into the interactions that are taken as evidence of engagement can inform both the domains that the staff are looking to implement and the domains in which interactions are occurring and their clarity.

For example, following self-harm, a practitioner will need to understand from the young person's perspective why they did it. The response by the young person may be 'I don't know', which is low domain clarity. However, as with the parent–young person interaction described earlier, the pacing and tone of voice and look, will be highly informative, as may the status of the practitioner. Equally important may be the aims of the practitioner when asking the question. Did the practitioner have Exploratory aims, or Safety aims? Does the interpretation of how engaged the young person is depend on the extent to which they are prepared to talk about their actions? The discussion of whether the young person is engaged (using the concept of the domains framework) thus becomes a discussion describing the way the practitioner aimed to interact and the responses that ensued.

The rapidly shifting moods and behaviours of young people in inpatient care are often problematic in some or all of these areas, and responses from nursing staff are quite likely to be domain unclear or mismatched. In this case an assessment along these dimensions has the potential to inform understanding of the disorder and the processes that undermine interactions within these inpatient settings.

Generally speaking, the practitioner (whether in a community or inpatient setting) can use the domains framework to formulate an understanding of the interactional processes between the young person and their parents. This can inform assessment and treatment aims. Likewise, the framework provides a means of understanding and improving communication between the practitioner and young person in inpatient settings. The domains framework can be used as a tool to help families understand that most families experience these types of difficulties, which will normalise their experience and reduce feelings of blame and guilt. The framework can also assist practitioners in inpatient settings to reduce the negativity inherent in difficult interactional processes, which often contribute to distress and behavioural difficulties.

Reflection

- How might you use the principles of the domains framework in your normal practice, when considering moment-by-moment interactions with your client group?

Conclusion

This chapter has offered a means of understanding moment-by-moment interaction in families and within practitioner–child therapeutic relationships. The domains framework offers a means of understanding and modifying interactions in order to improve meaning and clarity in daily communication. Creating a therapeutic alliance has been recognised as pivotal in the treatment of children's mental health. Emphasis on effective interpersonal therapeutic relationships relies upon a reciprocal process, with communication being positive, trusting and professional, with clear boundaries (Sergeant 2012). It is recognised and well documented within CAMHS nursing that the relationship is the key agent of change.

References

Anderson, H. & Gehart, D. (eds) (2007). *Collaborative Therapy: Relationships and Conversations that Make a Difference.* London: Routledge.

Association of Family Therapy (2016). *NICE Clinical Guidelines recommending Family and Couple Therapy.* https://www.aft.org.uk/SpringboardWebApp/userfiles/aft/file/NICE/NICE%20Clinical%20Guidelines%20recommending%20family%202016.pdf (last accessed 30.9.2019).

Bateson, G. (1972 [1964]). 'The logical categories of learning and communication.' In: G. Bateson (ed.) *Steps to an Ecology of Mind* (pp. 209-308). Chicago and London: University of Chicago Press.

Bolton, D. & Hill, J. (2004). *Mind, Meaning and Mental Disorder* (2nd edn). Oxford: Oxford University Press.

Bugental, D.B. (2000). Acquisition of the algorithms of social life: A domain-based approach. *Psychological Bulletin.* **126** (2), 187.

Byng-Hall, J. (2008). The crucial roles of attachments in family therapy. *Journal of Family Therapy.* **30**, 265-83.

Doane, J.A., Jones, J.E., Fisher, L., Ritzler, B., Singer, M.T. & Wynne, L.C. (1982). Parental communication deviance as a predictor of competence in children at risk for adult psychiatric disorder. *Family Process.* **21**, 211-23.

Epstein, N.B., Bishop, D.S. & Levin, S. (1978) The McMaster Model of Family Therapy Functioning. *Journal of Marriage and Family Counselling.* **4**, 19-31.

Fiske, A.P. (1992). The four elementary forms of sociality: framework for a unified theory of social relations. *Psychological Review.* **99**, 689-723.

Hill, J., Fonagy, P., Safier, E. & Sargent, J. (2003). The ecology of attachment in the family. *Family Process.* **42** (2), 205-21.

Hill, J., Pilkonis, P.A. & Bear, J. (2010). Social domains, personality and interpersonal functioning. In: L.M. Horowitz & S. Strack (eds) *Handbook of Interpersonal Psychology* (pp. 281-296). New York: Wiley.

Hill, J., Wren, B., Alderton, J., Burck, C., Kennedy, E., Senior, R., *et al.* (2014). The application of a domains-based analysis to family processes: implications for assessment and therapy. *Journal of Family Therapy.* **36** (1), 62-80.

Hutchings, J., Gardner, F., Bywater, T., Daley, D., Whitaker, C., Jones, K. *et al.* (2007) Parenting intervention in Sure Start services for children at risk of developing conduct disorder: pragmatic randomised controlled trial. *British Medical Journal.* **334**, 678.

Sergeant, A. (2012). *Working within Children & Adolescent Mental Health In-patient Services. A Practitioner's Handbook.* Available from: http://www.foundationpsa.org.uk/cms/upload_area/documents/Workingwithinchildandadolescentmentalhealthinpatientservices.pdf (last accessed 10.8.2019).

Stratton, P. (2016). *The Evidence Base of Family Therapy and Systemic Practice.* https://www.aft.org.uk/SpringboardWebApp/userfiles/aft/file/Research/Final%20evidence%20base.pdf (last accessed 30.9.2019).

Will, D. & Wrate, R.M. (1985). *Integrated Family Therapy.* London: Tavistock Publications Ltd.

Chapter 6

Perinatal mental health and working with families

Sue Barker

Introduction

'Childbirth is one of the most potent triggers for psychiatric illness' (Meltzer-Brody *et al.* 2018, p. 3). For many years, awareness of the potentially significant negative consequences for both the mother and the baby associated with maternal mental ill health has been increasing. There is now clear evidence that maternal suicide, due to mental illness, is a leading cause of maternal mortality in the UK, particularly perinatal mood disorders (Healthcare Quality Improvement Partnership 2017). Maternal mental health problems are also associated with an increased risk of low birthweight and premature birth, impaired mother–infant attachment and infant malnutrition during the first year of life (Meltzer-Brody *et al.* 2018).

One in four women experience perinatal mental health problems (Witcombe-Hayes *et al.* 2018); and one in ten fathers and other family members can also be affected (Melzer-Brody *et al.* 2018). In its 'All Babies Count' report, the National Society for the Prevention of Cruelty to Children (NSPCC) stated that, in England, approximately 122,000 babies under 1 year are living with a parent who has a mental illness. In the US, 6% of women experience depression in pregnancy and 11% in the first year after birth, whereas nearly 20% of women in developing countries experience symptoms of mental illness (Cluxton-Keller & Bruce 2018).

Maternal depression is a well-established health concern but more recently a strong link between maternal depression and paternal depression has been reported (Meltzer-Brody *et al.* 2018). The father's and mother's experiences are compounded by the bidirectional association between family relational stress and perinatal depression, in that lack of family support is both a predictor and a consequence of perinatal depression (Cluxton-Keller & Bruce 2018). There is growing evidence indicating that perinatal mental illness has a significant effect on children, especially on their growth and wellbeing, and this has led to a proliferation of policy development to reduce or ameliorate this experience.

Aims and learning outcomes

This chapter aims to examine the issues related to mental health during the perinatal period and to explore approaches that could be helpful to families during this time, applying a family-centred focus to a range of assessment and intervention processes. Having completed this chapter, the reader will:

- Have an understanding of the key issues that affect parents during the perinatal period
- Have an overview of some useful family-focused approaches to help families during this time.

Policy development

Women can experience the whole range of mental health problems in the perinatal period. In the most extreme cases, the most concerning outcome may be that the woman takes her own life. Sadly, the rate of maternal death by suicide has remained unchanged since 2003. Suicide is now identified as the main cause of maternal deaths occurring within a year after birth in the UK (Healthcare Quality Improvement Partnership 2017).

Policy responses to this began with the Department of Health (1999) highlighting postnatal depression as a priority within the National Service Framework (NSF) for Mental Health. Also, at this time, an independent evaluation of services by the Maternal Mental Health Alliance called 'Everyone's Business' became a key catalyst for change in perinatal mental healthcare (Granville *et al.* 2016). Yet, despite evaluation, campaigns and the publication of guidance, perinatal mental health continues to be a significant concern, and it was prominently featured, and additional funding was released, in the Next Steps in the Five-Year Forward NHS plan (NHS England 2017).

In England, developing services and improving outcomes for women with perinatal mental health problems and their families has been identified as a national priority. The UK Government ringfenced £365 million for NHS England's perinatal mental health community services development fund (between 2015/16 and 2020/21) (NHS England 2016). In Wales a review of the services available (in 'From Bumps to Babies') is currently influencing Welsh NHS policy (Witcombe-Hayes *et al.* 2018). Also, in 2018 Scotland set out its plan for perinatal mental healthcare on p. 64 of the 'Delivering for Today, Investing for Tomorrow, The Government's Programme for Scotland 2018–19' (Scottish Government, 2018) with Northern Ireland conducting a review of services in 2017.

It is anticipated that all women will eventually be able to access specialist mental health support from preconception through to a year after the birth of the baby in all areas of the UK. It is also recommended that fathers and the wider family should receive support.

Maternal perinatal mental health

In pregnancy and the postnatal period, women are vulnerable to having or developing the same range of mental health problems as at other times, such as depression, anxiety disorders, eating disorders, drug and alcohol use disorders, post traumatic stress disorder and severe mental illness (including psychosis, bipolar disorder, schizophrenia and severe depression). However, it is recognised that some changes in mental health state and functioning (such as appetite) may represent normal pregnancy changes, but they may also be symptoms of a mental health problem (NICE 2018).

Risk factors for developing a mental health problem in the perinatal period include a past history of depression, anxiety or bipolar disorder, as well as psychosocial factors, such as ongoing conflict with a partner, poor social support, and ongoing stressful life events (O'Hara *et al.* 2014). Women who have few social supports, poor health, a history of stressful life events and poor coping skills are at increased risk of poor mental health during the perinatal period (Stuart & Koleva 2014, Meltzer-Brody *et al.* 2018). These psychosocial factors are widely acknowledged but other factors have also been identified, which may have a negative impact on mental health. These include changes in auto-immune and hormonal levels, and genetic and epigenetic factors, in addition to circadian rhythm disruptions and sleep deprivation (Meltzer-Brody *et al.* 2018).

Perinatal mental illness can significantly affect the mother and infant relationship (Stuart & Koleva 2014), as perinatal mental disorders impair a woman's social functioning and they are associated with suboptimal development of her infant (O'Hara *et al.* 2014). Due to the potential negative impact on maternal and child outcomes, the perinatal period is a critical time to identify and treat mental illnesses (Paschetta *et al.* 2014).

Paternal perinatal mental health

In the past, perinatal mental health problems were viewed as gender specific; it was assumed that only women could experience perinatal mental ill health. Women were said to experience anorexia nervosa (the diagnosis included amenorrhea) and hysteria. However, it is now widely recognised that both mothers and fathers experience eating disorders and hysterical reactions. It should therefore be no surprise that men also develop perinatal mental ill health. A father's experience of perinatal mental health problems could be predicted by recognition of the monumental changes in life experiences they will be undergoing; they may struggle with their new role and identity, the competing challenges of fatherhood, negative feelings and fears, stress and lack of support (Baldwin *et al.* 2018).

Some of the coping strategies used by fathers include denial or escape activities, such as smoking, working longer hours or listening to music (Baldwin *et al.* 2018). Whilst these strategies can be useful in the short term, they do not help resolve the underlying issues. As with women, there are many barriers to men seeking and accepting support with their mental health at this time, and the most commonly recorded barrier is the stigma associated with mental illness. Other barriers for men include a lack of focused information resources and a lack of acknowledgment from healthcare professionals (Baldwin *et al.* 2018).

Paternal depression was very under-researched until the 21st century but there is now evidence suggesting that twice as many new fathers will experience depression as other men of the same age (Madsen & Burgess 2010). The causes identified for paternal mental ill health during the perinatal period are very similar to those recognised for women:

- Infant-related problems (e.g. frequent feeding, crying, etc.)
- Personality
- Previous mental ill health
- Lack of support
- Poor relationship with the mother
- Unemployment
- Unintended pregnancy.

There is some emerging research detailing the impact of paternal depression. Fathers can be less engaged and sensitive to their infant's needs, leading to developmental and behavioural problems exhibited by the children in a similar way to when mothers have depression (Fatherhood Institute 2010). Lack of engagement and sensitivity to the child by their main caregivers (usually their parents) can lead to attachment issues.

Family structures

Contemporary families can have quite diverse structures. In western society a baby may be brought up in a family with two mothers or two fathers, a mother and stepfather or vice versa; or the family may consist of one adult and other children, or they could be brought up in an adoptive family. Given the research now available on paternal perinatal mental health, practitioners should prepare themselves to offer support to the whole family, regardless of the family structure. Paternal perinatal mental illness research demonstrates that it can be triggered by psychosocial factors such as identity and relational changes.

Impact on child

Parental mental health problems can have monumental effects on the child. They can adversely affect cognitive, emotional, social, physical and behavioural development in both the short and long term (Cluxton-Keller & Bruce 2018, Meltzer-Brody et al. 2018). There is also an increased risk of psychopathology (Suarez et al. 2018). Between 25% and 50% of children who have a parent with a mental illness will experience some form of psychological disorder during childhood or adolescence, and 10% to 14% of these children will be diagnosed with a psychotic disorder at some point in their lives (van Doesum & Hosman 2007).

Research has also shown that untreated perinatal depression can adversely affect birth outcomes, result in poor maternal–infant interaction and increase the risk for child maltreatment (Cluxton- Keller & Bruce 2018). In addition, perinatal mood disorders are associated with an increased risk of low birthweight and premature birth, impaired mother–infant attachment and infant malnutrition during the first year of life (Meltzer-Brody et al. 2018).

A child who undergoes adverse life experiences is more likely to develop perinatal mental health problems themselves, which may lead to their children also experiencing poor attachments. Secure attachments in infancy are key predictors of positive neurological, psychological and social outcomes for the child (Meltzer-Brody et al. 2018). If provision is not in place for the family during the perinatal period and the issues of attachment are not addressed, the child is at high risk of adverse short- and long-term outcomes (Meltzer-Brody et al. 2018). Psychodynamic theorists, such as Bowlby, regard love, closeness and attachment as fundamental emotions, which are required for health and wellbeing (Bowlby 1952). Bowlby clearly states that infants who do not have secure attachments are likely to develop 'affectionless psychopathy', mental illness or become socially deviant (Bowlby 1952), and this premise appears to be upheld by contemporary research.

Attachment

Attachment describes a state in which the infant and mother are in a continuous relationship, where the infant experiences warmth and intimacy and both find satisfaction and enjoyment (Bowlby 1952). This theory of attachment developed over a number of years, and Bowlby later presented a model of how a lack of early attachment could have long-term effects on the person (Bowlby 1969). This was called the internal working model and it indicated that early life experiences could lead the infant to develop beliefs and expectations about the world and relationships. If the infant has received continuous love from its mother, it will develop the belief that people can be trusted, that they are worthy of love and that people care. The infant then carries this forward to future relationships, including their own parenting. These expectations lead to a perception of the world as being benevolent, which is self-reinforcing.

Evidence consistently demonstrates that the infants and children of women with high levels of distress, who are not able to develop this attachment, go on to have developmental and behavioural problems (Meltzer-Brody *et al.* 2018, Henshaw *et al.* 2009, McMahon *et al.* 2001, Lemaitre-Sillere 1998, Miller *et al.* 1993). Higher levels of aggression were also found to be expressed in children exposed to maternal depression (Hipwell *et al.* 2005). A mother with postnatal depression can have an impact on the whole family (Cluxton-Keller & Bruce 2018, Henshaw *et al.* 2009).

Whilst Bowlby's original theory viewed the mother–child relationship (monotropy) as the only one able to address the infant's attachment needs, it has since been established that the attachment needs of a baby can be fulfilled by the father or another close carer. The child can also have multiple attachments – it is not the number that is important but the quality of the relationship (Hanley 2009, Henshaw *et al.* 2009). Thus, those involved with women in the perinatal period can play a crucial role in reducing the risk of infants developing emotional and behavioural problems and support their developing wellbeing.

Perinatal assessment

Mental health problems are associated with personal and social stigma, which can reduce motivation for mothers and fathers to come forward for assessment and treatment. There is an extra concern for parents, as they may fear they will be considered 'unfit' and have their child removed (Leonard, Linden & Grant 2018). NICE (2014, updated 2018) provides clear guidance and standards of care, with one section of the guidance focused on assessment. It states that assessment and diagnosis of a suspected mental health problem in pregnancy and the postnatal period should include:

- History of any mental health problem, including in pregnancy or the postnatal period
- Physical wellbeing (including weight, smoking, nutrition and activity level) and history of any physical health problem
- Alcohol and drug misuse
- The woman's attitude towards the pregnancy, including denial of pregnancy
- The woman's experience of pregnancy and any problems experienced by her, the foetus or the baby
- The mother–baby relationship
- Any past or present treatment for a mental health problem, and response to any treatment
- Social networks and quality of interpersonal relationships

- Living conditions and social isolation
- Family history (first-degree relative) of mental health problems
- Domestic violence and abuse, sexual abuse, trauma or childhood maltreatment
- Housing, employment, economic and immigration status
- Responsibilities as a carer for other children and young people or other adults.

It is important that early recognition and referral to specialist care is arranged, whether the concerns are for the father or mother. There are a number of assessment tools available within mental health services such as the Patient Health Questionnaire 9, the Beck Depression Inventory for Primary Care, and the Hospital Anxiety and Depression Scale, but most commonly used is the Edinburgh Post Natal Depression Scale for women. There is some debate about the use of assessment tools such as the Edinburgh Post Natal Depression Scale but NICE (2014, updated 2018) offer the following guidelines.

At a woman's first contact with primary care or her booking visit, consider inviting her partner (and/or baby's father); and during the early postnatal period, consider asking the following depression identification questions as part of a general discussion about mental health and wellbeing:

- During the past month, have you often been bothered by feeling down, depressed or hopeless?
- During the past month, have you often been bothered by having little interest or pleasure in doing things?

Also consider asking about anxiety using the 2-item Generalized Anxiety Disorder scale (GAD-2):

- Over the last 2 weeks, how often have you been bothered by feeling nervous, anxious or on edge?
- Over the last 2 weeks, how often have you been bothered by not being able to stop or control worrying?

These are similar to the questions that NICE recommends asking anyone for whom there is a concern about low mood and/or anxiety. Whilst they may appear minimal and superficial, they do offer a starting point for discussion and the opportunity to explore whether there is a need for referral to mental health services. There are still differences in the availability of services, depending on geographical location. In a few areas in the UK there are inpatient facilities specifically for mothers and babies but in other areas the women and their families will be assessed and supported by the general community mental health team. Each team may use different assessment tools to assess the level of risk and which treatment approach may be most useful. The standard mental health assessment should allow practitioners to determine what the problems are and to develop a risk and treatment plan.

Given the level of risk and need for this client group, a multidisciplinary approach is essential. A midwife or health visitor will be allocated to each expectant mother, along with an obstetrician (depending on the woman's physical health needs), and it is important that both these healthcare professionals are kept informed of any risks and therapeutic interventions. It may also be necessary to involve social services and non-statutory agencies. It is crucial to co-ordinate care and ensure that all involved are kept informed. Depending on the level of need, medication will usually be prescribed by the GP or psychiatrist. In some areas there are nurse specialists who can undertake this role but if there is no requirement for medication a psychiatrist may not be part of the care team.

Interventions

The majority of preventive and treatment studies for perinatal depression are focused either on the mothers individually or on the mother–baby interaction (Cluxton-Keller & Bruce 2018). This continues to be the case, despite the developing recognition of paternal perinatal mental health problems. If fathers were better prepared and their relationships were supported, many fathers feel they would be more able to cope with the transition to parenthood, the outcomes would be more satisfactory and mental wellbeing would be enhanced (Baldwin *et al.* 2018). All mental health interventions, especially those related to perinatal mental health, should involve an element of psycho-education which could have a family focus; and the risks and benefits of each treatment should always be explained to the woman and her family (Meltzer-Brody *et al.* 2018). These needs fit well with family interventions and the recovery approach.

The recovery approach, which is now widely accepted, aims to recognise the unique life experiences of the parents and to build on the strengths they already possess. Identifying coping strategies they have found helpful in the past, and the social network available to them, will support their recovery journey. Likewise, based on a recovery assessment, problem-solving activities can enhance self-esteem, dignity and sense of control, which can lead to a sense of hope for the future.

Check the birth experience:

- Were there complications?
- Was it experienced as traumatic?

If the birth experience was identified as particularly challenging, the parents may need some time and space to talk to a health practitioner. The 'listening' visits by health visitors may be sufficient but if one of the parents is experiencing intrusive thoughts, flashbacks or nightmares they may have post-traumatic stress disorder (PTSD) which will require specialist treatment. NICE (2014, updated 2018) recommends Focused Cognitive Behavioural Therapy (FCBT) or Eye Movement Desensitisation and Reprocessing for PTSD during the perinatal period. Interpersonal therapy has also been found to be efficacious (Nillni *et al.* 2018).

Illustrative case study 1

Jack and Jennie have a six-week-old baby. They both felt shocked by the birth experience, with which they have mostly come to terms. However, they are both exhibiting symptoms of low mood and anxiety when their GP sees them at their six-week check-up. Jack states that Jennie's personality has changed since having the baby; he says she keeps crying and she no longer looks after herself or their home. Jennie states that Jack expects too much of her and keeps finding excuses not to take his share of housework and childcare. The GP refers them for couples' interpersonal therapy.

When they arrive for their first session, the therapy is explained to them and they agree to the aim of improving communication to enhance their relationship and their mental wellbeing. The practitioner initially gets Jack and Jennie to explain what their expectation of parenthood was, without interruption. They struggle not to argue with each other's description but afterwards agree that when they go home they will record times when they feel the other person is being unreasonable.

At the next session Jack and Jennie inform the practitioner that they have talked to each other about their expectations, and they have identified some expectations which they now realise are just fanciful. This has helped them feel more comfortable with each other. The practitioner then explores their records of when they believe their partner was being unreasonable. Most of the occasions were identified by both of them but some were recorded by only one partner.

Over the six sessions, the practitioner is able to facilitate Jack's and Jennie's recognition that they have both been trying to re-enact the way they themselves had been parented but Jack's parents fulfilled stereotypical gender roles and Jennie's parents did not. Jack and Jennie were helped to identify the type of relationship they wanted with each other and their baby. They developed coping strategies to help them problem-solve the new situations they found themselves in as the baby grew.

Observing parent–child interactions

Attachment is a key factor in the impact of parental mental ill heath on the infant and it can be assessed by observing the parent–child interaction. There are tools available to support healthcare practitioners in assessing sensitivity and improving attachment between parent and child. Whilst all tools have their limitations, the Neonatal

Behavioural Assessment Scale (NBAS) has been found to be useful with babies up to 3 months old and some health visitors use a video interactive guide.

Neonatal Behavioural Assessment Scale

The Neonatal Behavioural Assessment Scale (NBAS) is used to interpret a baby's signals and cues to help parents respond sensitively and develop attachments with their baby. It is also known as the Brazelton Neonatal Assessment Scale (BNAS). The NBAS tests newborn babies' abilities, usually when they are between 3 days and 4 weeks old but it can be used up to 3 months. It measures a variety of areas, including neurological, social and behavioural functioning, reflexes, responses to stress, startle reactions, cuddliness, motor maturity, ability to habituate to sensory stimuli, and hand–mouth coordination. This information is shared with parents to support their interactions.

With a Video Interactive Guide, the interactions of the parent and baby are recorded with a video device. The interactions are then discussed with the parent by the healthcare practitioner afterwards, to develop their sensitivity and attachment.

Review the feeding pattern of the baby/Explore sleep patterns and deprivation

A new mother and father may feel overwhelmed by their baby's need for frequent feeds and this may lead to sleep deprivation. This is an area that required detailed exploration, as nutrition and sleep are essential for mental and physical wellbeing for both the parents and baby. With social support, the parents may be able to develop their own routines that suit the whole family. However, they may need professional support with this if they are struggling with their mental health. A problem-solving approach (Pryjmachuk 2016) will be most useful.

Illustrative case study 2

Sam and Chris are becoming sleep deprived, as their baby Ali wakes and cries for food at less than two-hourly intervals throughout the night. This wakes both of them and, once they are awake, they find it difficult to return to sleep. The goal is for Sam, Chris and Ali to have sufficient food and sleep. Through a brainstorming approach, a number of options were discussed as follows:

- Another family member to care for and feed Ali once a week to allow Sam and Chris to catch up on sleep
- Sam and Chris to spend alternate nights in another family member's house to get a good night's sleep
- Sam and Chris to take turns to get up and feed Ali.
- Ali to be commenced on timed feeds.

Sam and Chris decided that the best option was for Sam's parents to care for Ali one night a week and for them to take turns in feeding Ali the rest of the week. They also decided to start a bedtime routine for the family so that they all felt prepared and ready for bed, to optimise sleep.

Approaches that might be adopted following a miscarriage or stillbirth

NICE (2014, updated 2018) offers the following guidance to reduce the risk of mental illness after miscarriage or stillbirth. These can be implemented with the immediate family, thus strengthening the family support and unity at this difficult time:

- Seeing a photograph of the baby
- Having mementos of the baby
- Seeing and holding the baby after the miscarriage or stillbirth.

This should be undertaken by an experienced practitioner, and the woman, her partner and family should be offered a follow-up appointment in primary or secondary care. A follow-up appointment should then be arranged, to see a midwife, nurse or GP in the GP surgery (primary care) or at the hospital with a midwife or obstetrician (secondary care) to establish whether the mother and family are developing healthy coping strategies and give them a chance to discuss any concerns that may have arisen due to miscarriage or stillbirth.

Illustrative case study 3

Mary was feeling a mixture of emotions when she was informed that her daughter was stillborn. Mary felt hurt and angry as well as terribly isolated and alone. She refused to see her dead daughter or give her a name. David felt numb and just accepted what the midwife and obstetrician suggested. David gave his daughter a cuddle and had his photograph taken with her. Mary was keen to leave hospital but they both accepted a follow-up appointment at the hospital.

At the follow-up appointment Mary was feeling low and a bit tearful but had framed the photo of David and Lilly (the name they had given their daughter). She was also carrying a copy around on her phone. At the appointment Mary and David were able to ask lots of questions such 'why did it happen?' and 'will it happen again?'

Family interventions

This chapter has outlined the impact perinatal mental illness can have on the whole family; and it is therefore reasonable to suggest that a whole family approach to interventions may be useful. Family-focused practice (FFP) is recommended for health visitors, and for nurses working with children and young people (Wright & Leahey 2013) and is therefore a good approach for perinatal practitioners as well. FFP can be defined as an umbrella term encompassing a continuum of family-focused care (Leonard, Linden & Grant 2018) and this approach has been adopted in most health and social care practices.

Family therapy is based on systems theory, which explores how family interactions affect each individual as well as their functioning as a whole family. Family therapy has also been found to be efficacious for the treatment of depression outside the perinatal period, particularly for young people and adults with depression. Research is now available which demonstrates the effectiveness of family intervention for the prevention and treatment of perinatal depression (Cluxton-Keller & Bruce 2018).

Family-focused therapeutic interventions are more specific, as they address relationship dynamics to create changes in relational functioning. This approach also covers: behavioural marital therapy, cognitive behavioural skills training, interpersonal therapy, and solution-focused therapy (Cluxton-Keller & Bruce 2018). Family interventions focus on improving communication skills between members of the family, including discussing their expectations of parenthood. The quality of parental relationships, particularly how parents communicate and relate to each other, is acknowledged as a primary influence on parenting and children's long-term mental health and future life chances. Family interventions can provide emotional support, and can also help develop problem-solving and conflict management skills. This is usually undertaken with a psycho-educational or cognitive behavioural therapy approach. These interventions can be provided in transition to parenthood programmes, which aim to facilitate healthy communication between parents, develop healthy family rules and limits, create shared responsibility in childrearing, and teach parenting skills to increase positive behaviour (Cluxton-Keller & Bruce 2018).

Children's programmes are one family-focused way of attempting to protect families, especially children, from the effects of perinatal mental ill health. Mental health services also provide family interventions through Child and Adolescent Mental Health Services (CAMHS) and Perinatal Mental Health Services (PMHS). These are secondary healthcare services that are normally accessed through the families' GP. However, some care pathways allow for referral by health visitors or midwives.

Reflection

- What do I understand about men's mental health during the perinatal period?
- How can care be family-focused in the postnatal period?

Conclusion

All the therapeutic interventions in this chapter are considered family interventions. As can be seen there is a continuum of interventions, some of which involve very basic relationship skills such as social support and problem-solving. NICE (2014, updated 2018) recommends a stepped approach to perinatal mental healthcare so parents with minor anxiety and mood problems may be supported by regular care from their health visitor and GP. Others, with more serious problems, may need to step up to more focused interventions such as listening visits, solution-focused therapy and problem-solving. People who have a diagnosis prior to pregnancy will need to be referred to their regular psychiatrist by the perinatal team. Those who experience a psychosis for the first time in the perinatal period need to be urgently referred to the perinatal team and they are likely to need hospital admission and medication.

Parents who experience significant mental health problems in the perinatal period are known to benefit from family interventions such as interpersonal therapy and problem-solving approaches.

Further reading

An excellent resource for healthcare professionals interested in perinatal mental health. http://www.rcgp.org.uk/clinical-and-research/resources/toolkits/perinatal-mental-health-toolkit.aspx (last accessed 11.8.2019).

References

Baldwin, S., Malone, M., Sandall, J. & Bick, D. (2018). Mental health and wellbeing during the transition to fatherhood: a systematic review of first time fathers' experiences. *The JBI Database of Systematic Reviews and Implementation Reports*. 2118–91.

Bowlby, J. (1952). Maternal care and mental health. *Journal of Consulting Psychology*. **16** (3), 232.

Bowlby, J. (1969). *Attachment. Attachment and loss: Vol. 1. Loss*. New York: Basic Books.

Cluxton-Keller, F. & Bruce, M.L. (2018). Clinical effectiveness of family therapeutic interventions in the prevention and treatment of perinatal depression: A systematic review and meta-analysis. *PLoS ONE*. **13** (6), e0198730. https://doi.org/10.1371/journal.pone.0198730 (last accessed 11.8.2019).

Department of Health (DH) (1999). *National Service Framework for Mental Health*. London: Department of Health.

Fatherhood Institute (2010). *Fathers and Postnatal Depression*. http://www.fatherhoodinstitute.org/2018/fatherhood-institute-research-summary-fathers-and-postnatal-depression/ (last accessed 11.8.2019).

Granville, G., Sugarman, W. & Tedder, V. (2016). *Maternal Mental Health Alliance 'Everyone's Business' Campaign. Independent Evaluation Report*. Gillian Granville Associates & WSA Community Consultants.

Hanley, J. (2009). *Perinatal Mental Health*. Chichester: Wiley Blackwell.

Healthcare Quality Improvement Partnership (HQIP) (2017). *MBRRAC-UK, Perinatal Confidential Enquiry*. London: HQIP.

Henshaw, C., Cox, J. & Barton, J. (2009). *Modern Management of Perinatal Psychiatric Disorders*. London: Royal College of Psychologists Publications.

Hipwell, A.E., Murray, L., Ducournau, P. & Stein, A. (2005). The effects of maternal depression and parental conflict on children's peer play. *Child: Care, Health & Development*. **31** (1), 11–23.

Lemaitre-Sillere, V. (1998). The infant with a depressed mother: destruction and creation. *Journal of Analytic Psychology*. **43**, 509–21.

Leonard, R.A., Linden, M. & Grant, A. (2018). Family-focused practice for families affected by maternal mental illness and substance misuse in home visiting: a qualitative systematic review. *Journal of Family Nursing*. **24** (2) 128–55.

Madsen, S.A. & Burgess, A. (2010). 'Fatherhood and mental health difficulties in the postnatal period' In: Conrad & White (eds) *Promoting Men's Mental Health*. Oxford: Radcliffe Publishing.

McMahon, C., Barnett, B., Kowalenko, N., Tennant, C. & Don, N. (2001). Postnatal depression, anxiety and unsettled infant behaviour. *Australian and New Zealand Journal of Psychiatry*. **35**, 581–88.

Meltzer-Brody, S., Howard, L.M., Bergink, V., Vigod, S., Jones, I., Munk-Olsen, T., Honikman, S. & Milgrom, S. (2018). Postpartum psychiatric disorders. *Nature Reviews, Disease Primers 4*. 18022. 1–18.

Miller, A.R., Barr, R.G. & Eaton, W.O. (1993). Crying and motor behaviour of six week old infants and post-partum maternal mood. *Paediatrics*. **92** (4), 551–58.

National Institute for Health and Care Excellence (NICE) (2014, updated 2018). *Antenatal and postnatal mental health: clinical management and service guidance*. https://www.nice.org.uk/guidance/CG192 (last accessed 11.8.2019).

NHS England (2016). *Perinatal.* https://www.england.nhs.uk/mental-health/perinatal/ (last accessed 11.8.2019).

NHS England (2017). *Next Steps on the NHS Forward View* https://www.england.nhs.uk/wp-content/uploads/2017/03/NEXT-STEPS-ON-THE-NHS-FIVE-YEAR-FORWARD-VIEW.pdf (last accessed 25.9.2019).

Nillni, Y.I., Mehralizade, A., Mayer, L. & Milanovic, S. (2018). Treatment of depression, anxiety and trauma related disorders during the perinatal period: A systematic review. *Clinical Psychology Review.* https://doi.org/10.1016/j.cpr.2018.06.004 (last accessed 11.8.2019).

O'Hara, M.W., Wisner, K.L., Asher, H. & Asher, M. (2014). Perinatal mental illness: Definition, description and aetiology. *Best Practice & Research Clinical Obstetrics and Gynaecology.* **28**, 3–12.

Paschetta, E., Berrisford, G., Coccia, F., Whitmore, J., Wood, M.G., Pretlove, S. & Ismail, K.M.K. (2014). Perinatal psychiatric disorders: an overview. *American Journal of Obstetrics & Gynecology.* 501–509.

Pryjmachuk, S. (2016). 'Using the skills of problem solving.' In: N. Evans & B. Hannigan (eds) *Therapeutic Skills for Mental Health Nurses.* London: Open University Press. ISBN: 9780335264407

Scottish Government (2018). *Delivering for Today, Investing for Tomorrow, The Government's Programme for Scotland 2018-19.* https://www.gov.scot/publications/delivering-today-investing-tomorrow-governments-programme-scotland-2018-19/ (last accessed 25.9.2019).

Stuart, S. & Koleva, H. (2014). Psychological treatments for perinatal depression. *Best Practice & Research Clinical Obstetrics and Gynaecology.* **28**, 61–70.

Suarez, A., Lahti, J., Czamara, D., Lahti-Pulkkinen, M., Knight, A.K., Girchenko, P. & Raikkonen, K. (2018). Maternal antenatal depression and child psychiatric problems. *Journal of the American Academy of Child and Adolescent Psychiatry.* **57** (5), 321–28.

van Doesum, K.T., Hosman, C.M., Riksen-Walraven, J.M. & Hoefnagels, C. (2007). Correlates of depressed mothers' sensitivity toward their infants: The role of maternal, child, and contextual characteristics. *Journal of the American Academy of Child and Adolescent Psychiatry.* **46**, 747–56.

Witcombe-Hayes, S., Jones, I., Gauci, P., Burns, J., Jones, S. & O'Leary, S. (2018). From Bumps to Babies: perinatal mental healthcare in Wales. Perinatal Mental Health in Wales project, a collaboration between NSPCC Cymru/Wales, National Centre for Mental Health (NCMH), Mind Cymru and Mental Health Foundation, with support from the Maternal Mental Health Alliance Everyone's Business Campaign.

Wright, L.M. & Leahey, M. (2013). *Nurses and Families: A Guide to Family Assessment and Intervention.* 6th edn. Philadelphia, PA: F. A. Davis.

Chapter 7

Family support and involvement in secure mental health services

Mick McKeown, Fiona Jones, Sue Stewart and Sheena Foster

Introduction

Latterly, there has been growing interest in offering better support to the families of people cared for in secure or forensic mental health services, and these concerns go back some thirty years. Collectively, we have been involved in a number of relevant projects, including early work to establish psychosocial approaches at Ashworth High Secure Hospital in the UK, a study of provision across secure units in Scotland, and a review of support and involvement for families in English secure services. Our work and wider research have highlighted some important points about what constitutes best practice in the field, some notable deficiencies and impediments to progress, and some indications as to future developments that could enable us to better meet the needs of family carers. In this chapter we will cover all three of these aspects and illustrate them with testimony grounded in personal experience of different aspects of the carer's role and interface with services.

We have also been involved in the study of service user involvement practices in secure settings. Interestingly, near the top of service users' concerns has been a desire for more effective involvement and support of visiting family members. Latterly these concerns have been reflected in Commissioning for Quality and Innovation (CQUIN) targets within the service-level contracting process. These initiatives chime with broader policy objectives such as those contained in the Triangle of Care (Worthington *et al.* 2013), though such general documents are typically silent on specific forensic issues for carers.

Aims and learning outcomes

The aim of this chapter is to offer an overview of the work we have been doing to better support families of people who access secure services. Having completed the chapter, the reader will:

- Have an appreciation of the lived experiences of secure care
- Understand some options for working with families in this context.

Our interest in this subject comes from diverse perspectives: two of us are parents whose sons are currently under the care of secure services; one of us was previously detained in secure units, experiencing difficulties maintaining contact with family and young children at the time; and one of us used to work in secure services and was involved in early attempts to improve the support and involvement of families. We have all been involved, in various ways, in researching the needs and experiences of family carers and the responses of service providers.

Policy and service developments

Across a number of settings, family carers express fairly common needs, and this is no different within the secure care context. When asked, family carers typically want three broad things: they wish to receive information about the service and their relative's progress; they need a mixture of emotional and practical support; and they want to be involved in their relative's care, including having input into important decisions. To a greater or lesser degree, these concerns are reflected in the research undertaken in forensic contexts to date and in various developments and innovations designed to meet these needs.

Research findings have consistently made the case for better support and involvement for families of forensic patients (see p. 86, 'Experiences of family carers in a secure context'). Indeed, there are some cogent reasons why better support should be provided. Firstly, like all families, they desire to act upon caring familial relationships, to be involved and supportive, even though they may need help to accomplish this effectively. Secondly, families are often an untapped source of information that would help formal services care better for their relatives.

Families also have needs and rights of their own, some of which are independent of the patient or service user. For example, families have a stake in the progress of their relative through the forensic system but may not always agree with decisions made by services; hence they ought (at the very least) to be consulted on key decisions, such as discharge. Family members may have been directly or indirectly victimised. They may struggle to comprehend the behaviour of their loved one, or the need for them to enter the mental health or criminal justice system. Conversely, they may have been the first to anticipate the need for a more assertive response from services, but their concerns may have been ignored or dismissed by practitioners. Researchers have also highlighted the practical and emotional burden of care for families in this context, including the fear of violence or the actual experience of assault at the hands of their family member.

The term 'forensic carer' has been coined to refer to the families and friends of individuals typically detained in secure units but also those under the care of community forensic services. However, the phrase is problematic, as neither of the constituent terms 'forensic' or 'carer' sits comfortably with the diverse group that is so defined. Relatives and friends may prefer to be known by their relationship (mother, father, brother, sister, partner) or find it difficult to take on board the notion of informal care-giving in the context of secure services that segregate individuals from their families and communities.

Moreover, certain staff within services may be uneasy ceding a designated caring role to family members when they see themselves as the frontline carers. The 'forensic' appellation, indicating the interface between mental health services and the criminal justice system, is not universally approved of, and does not necessarily apply to all secure units or all individuals. However, leaving aside all these questions of terminology, we contend that families and friends of people admitted to secure care have their own distinct needs and can, with appropriate involvement, make a significant positive contribution.

In fact we might argue for a change in the language used, to reflect a more positive view of family carers. Firstly, the term 'forensic carers' should in itself alert service providers to the fact that these carers need more specialised support than others, as their case has already reached the stage of needing criminal justice intervention with all the stress that this involves. Secondly, if these carers raise queries or express opinions about decisions proposed or taken by professionals, using the term 'carer's concern' might be a good way of flagging up problems as they arise. Such problems should always be noted by the professional, even if it is decided that further action is not needed. Thirdly, professionals sometimes have a knee-jerk reaction to family involvement, whereby they assume that a raising of concerns indicates that they are dealing with 'problem/abusive families'. Can we not introduce alternative terminology to recognise the positive contribution made by family involvement? Using the phrase 'involved families' would reinforce the fact that carers or families can be an asset to services.

The notion of documented carers' concerns is of interest in reinforcing accountability. We can see from most surveys of carers, including the Scottish Forensic Carers study (Ridley *et al.* 2014), that family carers may repeatedly raise concerns about the person they care for. Quite often such concerns are neither formally acknowledged nor documented. This means that when the same problem occurs it is again taken in isolation, and frustration continues for the carer, who can often predict a build-up of events that will eventually lead to crisis care or actually precipitate entry to the forensic system.

Various UK policy initiatives have been influential in motivating and sustaining developments in this area. Early examples include the Care Programme Approach (CPA) for organising case management, and more recently the Triangle of Care, which advocates more systematic support and involvement of families. Other drivers for change have been notable inquiries into care service failings, such as those at Ashworth High Secure Hospital in the 1990s. Initiatives to implement psychosocial interventions, including family therapy (which engendered waves of relevant staff training beginning in the 1990s), have also been influential. More recently, an emphasis on recovery as a holistic organising principle for mental healthcare has begun to include secure services promising more thorough consideration of the needs and involvement of families (Allen 2010, Drennan & Aldred 2012, Chandler *et al.* 2013, Machin & Repper 2013).

In one study of service user involvement practices across secure units in a single English region, actively engaged service users prioritised the need for similar patterns of involvement for family carers (McKeown *et al.* 2002). The National Secure Services Recovery and Outcomes Network (which is organised across nine English regions, involving staff and service users from their respective secure services in strategic discussions and sharing of best practice) has reinforced calls for better support and involvement of family carers. Our current study of family carers in the English secure estate has witnessed a call for the establishment of a similar network for carers.

What is it like to be a family carer in a secure context?

A number of published studies, commentaries and occasional first-hand testimony provide accounts of the experiences and needs of family carers. Notable issues raised are listed below.

Experiences of family carers in a secure context

● The challenge to support and contact posed by visiting institutions that are often situated lengthy distances from home (McKeown & McCann 1995, McCann *et al.* 1996, Canning *et al.* 2009, Absalom-Hornby *et al.* 2011a, 2011b). As many secure units have wide catchment areas, it is common for service users to be placed far from home, placing a burden of travel on family and friends who wish to maintain contact.

● The stress or burden of care arising from the forensic context, which may include fear of violence or troubled family relationships (MacInnes & Watson 2002, Tsang *et al.* 2002, Ferriter & Huband, 2003). Family members may indeed have been victimised or assaulted by their relative, but this need not mean that they wish to cease contact or involvement in care. Rather, such family members will have particular needs and wishes for appropriate service responses and support and these can often be left unmet. Such concerns extend to the desire to have a constructive say in discharge planning.

● The stress involved in dealing with services and security regimes (McKeown & McCann 1995, McCann *et al.* 1996, Hughes & Hughes 2000, Ferriter & Huband 2003, Finlay, Carruthers *et al.* 2018). The processes and paraphernalia of security, though necessary, can be off-putting and alienating for visitors to secure units.

- The stress connected to the actual offence that brought the person into secure care, and dealings with police or the courts, or anxieties flowing from negative media coverage of secure services. This might involve fears that one's relative will be abused by other patients or staff (McKeown & McCann 1995, McCann *et al.* 1996, Hughes & Hughes 2000).
- Despite all the stresses and strains of caring in the forensic context, admission can offer a degree of peace of mind for families, who now feel safe and secure in the knowledge that services are in place and taking responsibility for day-to-day care (Robinson *et al.* 2017).
- The stigma associated with both mental health and offending, which can include hostility from neighbours or the media (McKeown & McCann 1995, McCann *et al.* 1996, Hughes & Hughes 2000, Robinson *et al.* 2017).
- Various needs for high-quality information and communication with services (McCann *et al.* 1996, Hughes & Hughes 2000, MacInnes & Watson 2002, Canning *et al.* 2009, MacInnes *et al.* 2013). Many service providers now produce high-quality information in mixed media. There is a need to keep information up to date and revisit to check comprehension.
- How best to meet a family's practical and emotional support needs (McCann 1993, McCann *et al.* 1996, Hughes & Hughes 2000, MacInnes & Watson 2002, Canning *et al.* 2009). Many family members have experienced stress or, indeed, trauma during their relative's admission to secure services, but few receive offers of psychological support. In this situation, families can experience unmet needs in dealing with self-blame and guilt (Ferriter & Huband 2003).
- Uncertainties regarding how best to deal with their relative's mental health problems (McKeown & McCann 1995, McCann *et al.* 1996, Hughes & Hughes 2000). Families are often hungry for knowledge concerning mental health, services, and how best to help.
- Visiting times may be unduly stressful for all concerned (McCann *et al.* 1996). There is, hence, a need to provide support before and after visiting for both families and service users to assist communication during visits and reduce stress for everyone involved.
- Most of the research focus has been upon inpatient secure services, but many families are equally concerned about the quality and availability of community forensic support, and whilst involved with inpatient services may have anxieties about the future (Robinson *et al.* 2017).
- Relatives of particular groups of service users, such as those diagnosed with autism, have substantial problems ensuring their family members receive appropriate care in the secure care sector, and this generates particular stresses and grievances for these families (Larch 2016).

Family carers' previous experiences of psychiatry may have been unhelpful – and there may have been a lack of family involvement in key decisions. For example, early family warnings about risk might not have been acted upon (Hughes & Hughes 2000, Nordstrom et al. 2006, MacInnes et al. 2013, Ridley et al. 2014). At the other end of the care pathway, families might reasonably expect to be involved in discharge planning, with their views about the desirability, or not, of future accommodation and its location in relation to the family home being taken into account. Family carers often view staff as over-cautious in balancing service users' right to privacy with carers' rights to share in information (Gray et al. 2008, MacInnes & Watson 2002). Jubb and Shanley (2002) note the degree to which confidentiality sometimes operates as a justification for not sharing information and effectively excluding families. Szmukler and Holloway (2012) argue that there is often minimal need for this to be the case. Slade et al. (2007) offer useful commentary. Taken together, these concerns can result in continuing frustrations for families and friends in their dealings with services.

Sheena's story

Sheena's son has experienced admission to hospitals at different levels of security, and his journey has often been challenging for her as his mother. This has been complicated by the fact that she has also been a victim of her son's offending. However, her biggest issue has been frustration with the pace of progress through the system and not feeling appreciated or taken seriously by decision-makers:

> Society sees me as a victim and my son as a violent criminal. The simple truth for me is that I'm his mum, he was deeply unwell and committed a violent act that was totally against the person he is. Within secure services he's considered a mentally ill patient or a mentally disordered offender. It feels as if I'm also expected to see him like this. They look at me blankly when I say, 'He's one of the nicest people you'll ever meet and is considerate and thoughtful to anyone he meets. The problem is he expects people to treat him as he treats others and then he gets confused and that's when he becomes unwell.' I think I've been labelled delusional, over-protective and possibly in denial of his violence. I won't change my mind; I want them to work with the person I know but they continue to regard me with suspicion.

> Three years after his admittance to a High Secure Service, his psychiatrist proudly announced at a Tribunal. 'We know now that by nature he's not violent.' If I had been believed in the first place, perhaps he could have been moved through the service quicker. Instead I spent the next three years saying, 'The criteria for admission is being of grave or immediate danger to himself or others. Why is he still here? Can you give me an example of when he has been of grave or immediate danger to anyone?'

> He was never actually a problem within services and always fully co-operative, yet spent a further three years in a High Secure Service.

Reflection points
- How might services involve family members in matters of care planning or risk assessment in order to reduce some of the frustrations felt by Sheena here?
- What do you think services could do to improve the pace of progress through the system, and how might this become an aspect of how we communicate with families?

Types of support and services for carers in forensic settings

Several surveys of the support provided for families have found that an increasing interest in meeting carers' needs in general psychiatry has not necessarily been reflected in forensic psychiatry (Canning *et al.* 2009, Cormac *et al.* 2010, Geelan & Nickford 1999, MacInnes *et al.* 2013, Ridley *et al.* 2014). The most recent of these focused on Scotland, replicating Canning and colleagues' (2009) methodology and found similar numbers of patients in sustained contact with families, at around 40%, and similarly variable quantity and quality of family support provided by services (Ridley *et al.* 2014). A range of supportive interventions have been suggested to meet the needs of families, but these are seldom all available in one place. Such supportive interventions may include:

- A comprehensive information pack (Canning *et al.* 2009)
- Ongoing provision of information, including general information about the service and specific information germane to the family's relative and their progress through the system (Cormac *et al.* 2010, MacInnes & Watson 2002, MacInnes *et al.* 2013)
- Involving families in information exchange – getting information from families as well as providing it for them (Cordess 1992, McCann & McKeown 1995)
- Regular events (Canning *et al.* 2009)
- Carers' support groups (McCann 1993)
- Dedicated staff focused on carer support, responsible for innovation and point of contact for new carers
- Welcome meetings soon after a person is admitted (Dimond & Chiweda 2011)
- Improved visiting arrangements, comfortable rooms and toys for children (see Cormac *et al.* 2010). Support with costs of visiting or assistance finding local overnight accommodation or provision on-site.
- Facilitating telephone contact (Ridley *et al.* 2014).

A particular issue within secure services is the complexity of keeping in touch with children. Progressive services make judicious attempts to maintain or re-initiate contact with service users' children (Chao & Kuti 2009) but changing concerns surrounding security and children's welfare can raise barriers to ongoing contact (see Fallon 1999). Fiona, a co-author of this chapter, experienced a not untypical dislocation from her children whilst detained in secure care, which was eventually resolved on discharge through sensitive and consensual re-engagement with her now adult family.

Fiona's story: The impact of secure care on families and children

When I was transferred from prison to high secure care, the first thing I noticed was the different rules around contact with children. Even though visiting in prison had been as simple as sending a visiting order and then waiting to go into the visiting hall, in secure care a whole new risk assessment had to be done by social workers. I had to put people on a list that I wanted to contact so I could no longer phone my children when I wanted, or write to them. I understood the risks about my children seeing some of the other patients but I felt like I was being doubly punished for being ill. All of a sudden I was 'untrustworthy' and 'to be viewed with suspicion'.

Eventually, social workers went to my parent's house to ask my son if he would like to see me. Of course he wanted to, but by then we hadn't seen each other for about 18 months. Long enough for my entire physical appearance to have changed and for me to be 'slowed down' by medication in speech, thought, effort.

The day of the first visit came. To be held away from the ward, in the company of several burly nurses dressed in black trousers and white shirts, key chains visible, walkie-talkies talking about 'movements' and 'escorts'. My parents and son were escorted into the room where I was sat. My mum and dad looked visibly shaken. I had no idea of the security checks and gates they'd had to walk through. And when they saw me, they looked defeated. I said 'hello son'. He looked around the room and saw me. He never said anything at the time, he just ran over and hugged me.

Many years later, he said the only thing he remembered about high secure was that day, walking through lots of gates, the sniffer dogs, the scanners and how he looked at me that day and thought 'someone has eaten my mum'. I was three times the size I had been when I last saw him (because of medication induced weight gain).

The impact on my daughter was greater in a lot of ways. We didn't see each other for five years. It was deemed 'in her best interests' to withhold all the letters I had written her and refuse phone calls. Her dad had died at the beginning of my sentence and she had lost her mum for a long time too (whilst my son was looked after by my parents, my daughter had been fostered out of my family). When we eventually met up again, she was angry. She had been angry with me for so long about not keeping in touch. Then, when she found out I had been trying and she got to read all the letters, she became angry with services.

Thankfully, today is a different story and I am in daily contact with both kids. My son came back to live with me and eventually so did my daughter. I am the proud

> nana of one lovely grandchild. What would have been helpful for my family would have been a bit of information about what was going to happen with regards to security practices, perhaps a warning about the wall, fences, gates. Wouldn't it have been kinder to my family to see 'nurses' in normal clothes without the obvious big dangly key chain, the alarms, the walkie talkies? I would have wanted someone to explain about my physical appearance and affect. Even showing a photograph or a family-friendly leaflet explaining that I might not be able to talk very well or move very fast. I might accidentally dribble or nod off. I would have liked someone to talk to my daughter and explain that I wasn't very well but that we could write to each other or phone. She hated me for years, thinking I had just 'gone away' and she'd done something wrong to end up in foster care.
>
> My family did not need to go through this to see their remnants of a daughter and mum. Communication and a bit of sensitivity could have made this less traumatic for them.

When we think about family connections, we might also reflect on how to help families by offering interventions that include the whole family, or at least those willing to take part. The next section considers such approaches.

Psychosocial interventions and family therapy

Broadly speaking, the term 'psychosocial interventions' (PSIs) refers to ways of organising and delivering care that are framed by case management principles and supported by effective provision of information and education. PSIs deliver packages of therapy that include both individual and family-focused behavioural and cognitive-behavioural interventions. Assorted research studies have demonstrated the value of this approach in general community settings, as indicated by reduced relapse rates and burden for relatives (Pharoah *et al.* 2010). Implementation approaches have built upon this research base, and involved mass practitioner training programmes, commencing in the 1990s with the Thorn initiative. Since then, various practitioners and researchers have sought to translate these initiatives into secure settings. The psychosocial stress arising in close interpersonal relationships is identified as significantly influential and open to amelioration through therapeutic work that targets the social network (usually the family), rather than being restricted to the individual.

Psycho-education approaches typically engage service users and/or carers in one-to-one or group learning about mental health and the service context to promote mutual self-help and support-seeking or better equip them to negotiate the care system (Mannion *et al.* 1994, Pekkala & Merinder 2002). Evaluations of psycho-education have demonstrated beneficial effects in secure settings, with service users alone (Aho-Mustonen *et al.* 2008, 2009, Vallentine *et al.* 2010, Walker *et al.* 2012, 2013) or carers alone (McCann, McKeown & Porter 1996). Though authors such as Klimitz (2006) argue it is best for psycho-education to involve carers and service users together, this might not always be feasible in secure environments, especially if the individual's offending involved victimising a member of the family (Vallentine et al. 2010). Despite general evidence of the value of psycho-education, its impact on service user outcomes (such as relapse) is thought to be limited unless it is delivered in conjunction with more systematic interventions, such as family therapy (Fadden 1998, Tarrier et al. 1998).

The most commonly undertaken psychosocial family support offered in Geelan and Nickford's (1999) survey of forensic units was psycho-education. An early study at Ashworth High Secure Hospital (McCann, McKeown & Porter 1996, McCann & Clancy 1996) found that providing information for carers, tailored to the high secure setting and supplemented with support group work and psycho-education, was beneficial and appreciated by family carers. Around this time, a psycho-education programme was implemented in Australian community settings where families were caring for individuals with forensic histories. In this initiative, aimed at preventing relapse or reoffending, the psycho-education component was combined with emotional and practical support. Latterly, psycho-education approaches have become more widespread within secure units, yet evaluative research lags behind (Nagi & Davies 2015).

The earliest programmatic attempt to implement and study PSI in secure settings was undertaken by McCann and colleagues at Ashworth High Secure Hospital in the 1990s (McKeown & McCann 1995, McCann & McKeown 1995, McCann, McKeown & Porter 1996, McCann & Clancy 1996, McKeown & McCann 1999, McCann & McKeown 2000). However, despite promising research findings and a degree of institutional support, this programme of work was ultimately undone due to organisational inertia (McKeown 2007).

A notable feature of secure settings is that, while service users are separated from family carers for extended periods of time, they spend large portions of time relating to staff. On the rare occasions when service users do meet family members, substantial psychosocial stresses are often at play, reinforcing the need to provide appropriate support. Visiting times can provoke raw emotions and become highly charged, with participants anxious not to say the 'wrong' thing to each other. This can stifle constructive communication, with families skirting round or avoiding talking about things that are important to them for fear of causing upset or prompting a negative reaction. Alternatively, or even simultaneously, well-meaning attempts at such communication may be enacted clumsily with the same stressful results (McKeown & McCann 1995, McCann, McKeown & Porter 1996). Certain fairly simple supportive interventions can help relatives better negotiate these potentially stressful encounters, helping them to cope with stress and leading to more fulfilling visits.

In the last two decades there have been various attempts to progress psychosocial practice developments within forensic settings. These endeavours have included initiatives with different client groups and at different levels of security: inpatient and community forensic services, psychiatric intensive care units (PICUs, or IPCUs in Scotland), learning difficulties services, dual-diagnosis services, forensic child and adolescent mental health services (CAMHS) (Savage & McKeown 1997, MacInnes 2000, Baker *et al.* 2002, Walker 2004, Isherwood *et al.* 2004, Gleeson *et al.* 2006, Lawless 2008, Peddie 2009, Atchinson *et al.* 2009, Richards *et al.* 2009, Absalom-Hornby *et al.* 2010). In one of the more ambitious programmes, Walker (2004) describes the adoption of PSI practices in the State Hospital at Carstairs.

More recently, Absalom-Hornby and colleagues in the North-West of England have reported on a range of relevant and innovative practices. This team have used digital technologies to support family therapy with families who cannot visit frequently because of distance (Absalom *et al.* 2010, Absalom-Hornby *et al.* 2011a, Absalom-Hornby *et al.* 2011b, Absalom-Hornby *et al.* 2012). Families found the use of web cameras to be an acceptable and helpful means of experiencing sophisticated psychosocial support, and positive social, emotional and practical outcomes were achieved (Absalom-Hornby *et al.* 2012). The same authors surveyed 11 wards in the region, comprising different levels of security. Despite over 70% of service users experiencing high levels of contact with their families, only 18% of services provided any type of family intervention (Absalom-Hornby *et al.* 2010). Such findings are typical in the literature, which generally shows minimal formal family interventions alongside patchy provision of information regarding diagnosis or treatment, amounting to a failure to meet relevant NICE standards (Gough *et al.* 2007).

Perhaps surprisingly, given the roots of PSI in general community services, forensic community services are somewhat under-represented in the literature regarding family carers. Within mainstream adult community mental health services, Gleeson *et al.* (2006) make recommendations for the adoption of a model of preventive forensic PSI to better meet the needs of individuals with a history of offending. McKeown (2001) presents a single case study of successful family work in the context of a person who has recently been discharged following a lengthy 'revolving-door' history of detention in secure units or prison settings. Positive outcomes included general improvements to well-being, reduced illicit drug consumption and associated criminality, and reduced psychosocial stress within the family.

Recent studies have shown increased provision of family therapy within secure services. In one survey, a third of responding medium secure units offered such intervention, with a preference for systemic approaches (Davies *et al.* 2014). In our own study of all English secure units, nearly 45% of service responses indicated the availability of family therapy, though this does not necessarily mean that large numbers of families are accessing it.

Case management and risk assessment

Generally speaking, mental health policy urges holistic models of case management and care coordination that typically ought to involve families (Hervey & Ramsay 2004, Wallcraft et al. 2011), and this policy rhetoric extends to family carers who are involved in caring for forensic patients (NIMHE 2004). Universal requirements to undertake carers' assessments or involve carers in discharge planning could be neatly accommodated within policy goals of collaboration, partnership and risk minimisation (see Simons et al. 2002, Rapaport et al. 2007). In the forensic context in particular, this opens up interesting debates about risk assessment, management and community re-integration, with a case being made for family carers becoming more substantially involved and, indeed, being viewed as a significant resource (Coffey 2012, McCann & McKeown 2002, Nordstrom et al. 2006). In general community settings, family carers recognise a number of ways in which they already informally attend to risk (Ryan 2002). Kennedy (2002) proposes a stratified system for risk management that acknowledges different levels of security and values supportive family involvement.

Irish commentators have suggested that an Integrated Care Pathway can shift services away from their traditional emphasis on security and towards more recovery-oriented approaches which support enhanced service user and carer involvement in identifying and understanding risks (Gill et al. 2010). Kelly et al. (2002) position carers as key partners in drawing up and applying risk management plans in the context of Australian community forensic care.

Open dialogue: New horizons for democratic involvement?

The open dialogue approach, developed in Finland but now spreading in influence, is founded on a systemic approach to supporting and intervening in people's social networks – typically the family context (Seikkula & Olson 2003). It also draws upon Bakhtin's (1984) social theory to make sense of the importance of the 'polyphonic' dialogue in this context. In a novel departure from mainstream approaches to care, this labour-intensive therapy adheres to some key principles, not least a commitment to speak openly and honestly in front of all present. Indeed, everything said is for the ears of the whole network; nothing is to be said outside family/network meetings. There is also a strong emphasis on the intelligibility of the individual's experiences – looking for 'meaning in madness' even if it is not immediately apparent. The approach is implicitly and explicitly democratic and dialogic, and as such is a departure from paternalistic bio-psychiatry. Attempts are also made to use medication sparingly.

Some outstanding results have been claimed for the open dialogue approach (and its precursor Needs Adapted Therapy), which has essentially been running for more than two decades as a large natural experiment in Western Lapland, with a number of formal research evaluations also undertaken (Aaltonen et al. 2011). Findings suggest that outcomes for service users are superior to those gained using other western psychiatric systems, and that second episodes of psychosis can be avoided with a concerted open dialogue intervention at the first episode. A number of key social outcomes, such as gainful employment, have been achieved with substantially large numbers of service users; while significantly lower numbers of individuals end up taking anti-psychotic prescriptions. Despite such positive findings, and sterling efforts at promotion of these ideas by the Open Dialogue UK organisation, many UK practitioners and service users are still unaware of the approach. Organised survivor groups are much more aware, and many are passionate campaigners for the adoption of this approach by mainstream services.

It could be argued that open dialogue techniques have much to offer forensic services: opening up opportunities to consider how best to involve the service user's social networks in both therapeutic support and risk assessment and management.

Reflection

- What do you think are the lessons for services about family relationships when a parent is admitted to secure services?
- How might we think about organising visits in secure care to make them more family-friendly?
- What are the important issues when balancing safeguarding and a right to family life?

Conclusion

Despite notable improvements in involving and supporting family carers with relatives in secure services, it is chastening to recall that the first Ashworth Public Inquiry, led by Louis Blom-Cooper (Department of Health 1992, p. 233), observed '… regrettably, the regime at Ashworth… seems to have been designed to deter rather than encourage relatives to participate in their relatives' care.'

We may pose the question, to what extent has this state of affairs comprehensively improved across secure services? Or, indeed, why has it taken so long to make adequate progress (where we can find it)? Collectively we have the wit and imagination to do so much better. There is ample evidence that some secure care services can and do provide a range of support and involvement initiatives for family carers, and that some of these are truly innovative and well-received. The main question is why so few services seem able to offer the complete range of initiatives to a high standard. Furthermore, it is disappointingly true that relatives who may have already been traumatised by the events leading up to their family member's admission to secure services often continue to find themselves equally traumatised by the system itself.

There is substantial scope to improve service responses to the demands and needs of family carers. If new developments, like Open Dialogue, can capture the zeitgeist by democratising the social relations of care, their implementation within the secure care context could represent a major step in the reform of these institutions. Greater democracy is implicit in policies that make a virtue of attending to service user, carer and staff voices alike. Applying such policies, at both the strategic and practice levels, could make holistic care a reality, as in the Triangle of Care. To achieve this within secure care services might, for once, place this often-maligned sector in the vanguard of transformative change, rather than lagging behind.

References

Aaltonen, J., Seikkula, J. & Lehtinen, K. (2011). The comprehensive open-dialogue approach in Western Lapland: I. The incidence of non-affective psychosis and prodromal states. *Psychosis.* **3** (3), 179–91.

Absalom, V., McGovern, J., Gooding, P. & Tarrier, N. (2010). An assessment of patient need for family intervention in forensic health services and staff skill in implementing family interventions. *Journal of Forensic Psychiatry and Psychology.* **21** (3), 350–65.

Absalom-Hornby, V., Gooding, P. & Tarrier, N. (2011a). Coping with schizophrenia in forensic health services: the needs of relatives. *Journal of Nervous and Mental Disease.* **199**, 398–402.

Absalom-Hornby, V., Gooding, P. & Tarrier, N. (2011b). Implementing family intervention within forensic health services: the perspectives of clinical staff. *Journal of Mental Health.* **20** (4), 355–67.

Absalom-Hornby, V., Hare, D., Gooding, P. & Tarrier, N. (2012). Attitudes of relatives and staff towards family intervention in forensic health services using Q methodology. *Journal of Psychiatric and Mental Health Nursing.* **19**, 162–73.

Absalom-Hornby, V., Gooding, P. & Tarrier, N. (2012). Family intervention using a web camera (e-FFI) within forensic health services: a case study and feasibility study. *The British Journal of Forensic Practice.* **14** (1), 60–71.

Aho-Mustonen, K., Miettinen, R., Koivisto, H., Timonen, T. & Raty, H. (2008). Group psycho-education for forensic and dangerous non-forensic long-term patients with schizophrenia: a pilot study. *European Journal of Psychiatry.* **22** (2), 84–92.

Aho-Mustonen, K., Miettinen, R. & Timonen, T. (2009). Experienced long term benefits of group psycho-education among forensic and challenging non-forensic patients with schizophrenia. *International Journal of Psychosocial Rehabilitation.* **14** (1), 51–63.

Allen, S. (2010). *Our Stories: Moving On, Recovery and Well-Being.* London: South West London & St George's Mental Health Trust Forensic Health Services.

Atchinson, M., Ginty, M. & Close, J. (2009). The Tuesday group: adapting family work within an inpatient child and adolescent mental health forensic health service. *Meriden: the West Midlands Behavioural Family Programme Magazine.* **3** (9), 12–14.

Baker, J., O'Higgins, H., Parkinson, J. & Tracey, N. (2002). The construction and implementation of a psychosocial interventions care pathway within a low secure environment: a pilot study. *Journal of Psychiatric & Mental Health Nursing.* **9**, 737–39.

Bakhtin, M. (1984). *Problems of Dostojevskij's Poetics.* Manchester: Manchester University Press.

Canning, A., O'Reilly, S., Wressell, L., Cannon, D. & Walker, J. (2009). A survey exploring the provision of informal carers' support in medium and high secure services in England and Wales. *The Journal of Forensic Psychiatry and Psychology.* **20**, 868–85.

Chandler, R., Bradstreet, S. & Hayward, M. (2013). *Voicing Caregiver Experiences: Wellbeing and Recovery Narratives for Caregivers.* Sussex Partnership NHS Foundation Trust/Scottish Recovery Network: Creative Commons.

Chao, O. & Kuti, G. (2009). Supporting children of forensic in-patients: whose role is it? *Psychiatric Bulletin.* **33**, 55–57.

Coffey, M. (2012). A risk worth taking? Value differences and alternative risk constructions in accounts given by patients and their community workers following conditional discharge from forensic mental health services. *Health, Risk & Society.* **14** (5), 465–82.

Cordess, C. (1992). *Family therapy with psychotic offenders and family victims in a forensic psychiatry secure setting. Proceedings of the 17th International Congress of the International Academy of Law and Mental Health.* Leuven, Belgium, 26–30 May 1991. International Academy of Law and Mental Health.

Cormac, I., Lindon, D., Jones, H., Gedeon, T. & Ferriter, M. (2010). Facilities for informal carers of in-patients in forensic psychiatric services in England and Wales. *The Psychiatrist.* **34**, 381–84.

Davies, A., Mallows, L., Easton, R., Morrey, A. & Wood, F. (2014). A survey of the provision of family therapy in medium secure units in Wales and England. *The Journal of Forensic Psychiatry and Psychology.* **25**, 520–34.

Department of Health (1992). *Report of the Committee of Inquiry into Complaints about Ashworth Hospital.* Cm 2028-1. Vols I and II. London: HMSO.

Dimond, C. & Chiweda, D. (2011). Developing a therapeutic model in a secure forensic adolescent unit. *Journal of Forensic Psychiatry and Psychology.* **22** (2), 283–305.

Drennan, G. & Aldred, D. (2012). *Secure Recovery: Approaches to Recovery in Secure Mental Health Settings.* London: Routledge.

Fadden, G. (1998). Research update: psycho-educational family interventions. *Journal of Family Therapy.* **20**, 293–309.

Fallon, P. (1999). *Report of the Committee of Inquiry into the Personality Disorder Unit, Ashworth Special Hospital.* https://www.gov.uk/government/publications/ashworth-special-hospital-report-of-the-committee-of-inquiry (last accessed 26.8.2019).

Ferriter, M. & Huband, N. (2003). Experiences of parents with a son or daughter suffering from schizophrenia. *Journal of Psychiatric and Mental Health Nursing.* **10**, 552–60.

Finlay-Carruthers, G., Davies, J., Ferguson, J. & Browne, K. (2018). Taking parents seriously: The experiences of parents with a son or daughter in adult medium secure forensic mental health care. *International Journal of Mental Health Nursing.* **27**. 10.1111/inm.12455.

Geelan, S. & Nickford, C. (1999). A survey of the use of family therapy in medium secure units in England and Wales. *Journal of Forensic Psychiatry and Psychology.* **10** (2), 317–24.

Gill, P., McKenna, P., O'Neill, H., Thompson, J. & Timmons, D. (2010). Pillars and pathways: foundations of recovery in Irish forensic mental healthcare. *British Journal of Forensic Practice.* **12** (3), 29–36.

Gleeson, J., Nathan, P. & Bradley, G. (2006). The need for the development and evaluation of preventative psychosocial forensic interventions in mainstream adult community mental health services. *Australasian Psychiatry.* **14** (2), 180–85.

Gough, K., Churchward, S., Dorkins, E., Fee, J., Oxborrow, S., Parker, J. & Smith, H. (2007). Audit of the NICE guidelines for schizophrenia in an NHS forensic psychiatric service. *The British Journal of Forensic Practice.* **9** (4), 28–34.

Gray, B., Robinson, C., Seddon, D. & Roberts, A. (2008). 'Confidentiality smokescreens' and informal carers for people with mental health problems: the perspectives of professionals. *Health and Social Care in the Community.* **16**, 378–87.

Hervey, N. & Ramsay, R. (2004). Carers as partners in care. *Advances in Psychiatric Treatment.* **10**, 81–84.

HM Government (2010). *Recognised, Valued and Supported: Next steps for the carers strategy.* London: Department of Health. https://www.gov.uk/government/publications/recognised-valued-and-supported-next-steps-for-the-carers-strategy (last accessed 26.8.2019).

Hughes, J. & Hughes, C. (2000). 'Family and friends.' In: D. Mercer, T. Mason, M. McKeown & G. McCann (eds) *Forensic Mental Healthcare: A Case Study Approach.* Edinburgh: Churchill Livingstone.

Isherwood, T., Burns, M. & Rigby, G. (2004). Psychosocial interventions in a medium secure unit for people with learning disabilities: a service development. *Mental Health and Learning Disabilities Research and Practice.* **1** (1), 29–35.

Jubb, M. & Shanley, E. (2002). Family involvement: the key to opening locked wards and closed minds. *International Journal of Mental Health Nursing.* **11** (1), 47–53.

Kelly, T., Simmons, W. & Gregory, E. (2002). Risk assessment and management: a community forensic practice model. *International Journal of Mental Health Nursing.* **11** (4), 206–13.

Kennedy, H. (2002). Therapeutic uses of security: mapping forensic mental health services by stratifying risk. *Advances in Psychiatric Treatment.* **8**, 433–43.

Klimitz, H. (2006). Psychoeducation in schizophrenic disorders – psychotherapy or 'infiltration'? *Psychiatric Practice.* **33**, 379–82.

Larch, S. (2016). Autism, mental health and offending behaviour: a mother's quest for healthcare. *Advances in Autism.* **2** (4), 210–214.

Lawless, S. (2008). *Social Work in a Psychiatric Intensive Care Unit and the Forensic Liaison Service with a focus on family interventions.* Conference paper: June 11th 2008. CRSI-Cork with University College Cork. Promoting Social Inclusion in Mental Health.

Machin, K. & Repper, J. (2013). *Recovery: a carers' perspective.* Centre for Mental Health & Mental Health Network, NHS Confederation.

MacInnes, D. (2000). Interventions in forensic psychiatry: the caregiver's perspective. *British Journal of Nursing.* **9** (15), 992–98.

MacInnes, D., Beer, D., Reynolds, K. & Kinane, C. (2013). Carers of forensic mental health in-patients: what factors influence their satisfaction with services? *Journal of Mental Health.* **22**, 528–35.

MacInnes, D. & Watson, J. (2002). The differences in perceived burden between forensic and non-forensic caregivers of individuals suffering from schizophrenia. *Journal of Mental Health.* **11** (4), 375–88.

Mannion, E., Mueser, K. & Solomon, P. (1994). Designing psychoeducational services for spouses of persons with serious mental illness. *Community Mental Health Journal.* **30** (2), 177–90.

Marshall, B. & Solomon, P. (2000) Releasing information to families of persons with severe mental illness: a survey of NAMI members. *Psychiatric Services.* **51**, 1006–1011.

McCann, G. (1993). Relatives' support groups in a special hospital: an evaluation study. *Journal of Advanced Nursing.* **18**, 1883–88.

McCann, G. & Clancy, B. (1996). Family matters. *Nursing Times.* **14** (7), 46–48.

McCann, G. & McKeown, M. (1995). Applying psychosocial interventions within a forensic environment. *Psychiatric Care.* **2**, 133–36.

McCann, G. & McKeown, M. (2000). 'Severe and enduring mental health problems: family work.' In: Mercer, D., Mason, T., McKeown, M. & McCann, G. (eds) (2000) *Forensic Mental Healthcare: A Case Study Approach.* Edinburgh: Churchill Livingstone. 91–98.

McCann, G. & McKeown, M. (2002). 'Risk and serious mental health issues.' In: N. Harris, S. Williams & T. Bradshaw (eds) (2002). *Psychosocial Interventions for People with Schizophrenia: A Practical Guide for Mental Health Workers.* Basingstoke: Palgrave-Macmillan, 205–210.

McCann, G., McKeown, M. & Porter, I. (1995). Identifying the needs of the relatives of forensic patients. *Nursing Times.* **91** (24), 35–37.

McCann, G., McKeown, M. & Porter, I. (1996). Understanding the needs of relatives of patients within a special hospital for mentally disordered offenders: a basis for improved services. *Journal of Advanced Nursing.* **23**, 346–52.

McKeown, M. (2001). 'Psychosocial interventions for a person with serious mental health problems, using street drugs, with a history of related offending.' In: G. Landsberg & A. Smiley (eds) (2001). *Forensic Mental Health: Working with Offenders with Mental Illness.* New Jersey: Civic Research Institute, **8**, 2–10.

McKeown, M. (2007). 'Psychosocial interventions at Ashworth: an occupational delusion.' In: D. Pilgrim (ed.) *Inside Ashworth: Professional Accounts of Institutional Life.* Oxford: Radcliffe Publishing, 59–80.

McKeown, M. & McCann, G. (1995). A schedule for assessing relatives: the relative assessment interview for schizophrenia in a secure environment. *Psychiatric Care.* **2** (3), 84–88.

McKeown, M. & McCann, G. (1999). 'Psychosocial interventions.' In: C. Chaloner & M. Coffey (eds) *Forensic Mental Health Nursing: Current Approaches.* Oxford: Blackwell Science, 232–51.

McKeown, M., McCann, G. & Forster, J. (2002). 'Psychosocial interventions in institutional settings.' In: N. Harris, S. Williams & T. Bradshaw (eds). *Psychosocial Interventions for People with Schizophrenia: A Practical Guide for Mental Health Workers.* Basingstoke: Palgrave-Macmillan, 211–35.

Nagi, C. & Davies J. (2015) Bridging the gap: brief family psychoeducation in forensic mental health, *Journal of Forensic Psychology Practice.* **15** (2), 171–183, DOI: 10.1080/15228932.2015.1013786

National Institute for Mental Health England (NIMHE) (2004). *Cases for Change: Forensic Mental Health Services.* London: NIMHE.

Nordstrom, A., Kullgren, G. & Dahlgren, L. (2006). Schizophrenia and violent crime: the experience of parents. *International Journal of Law and Psychiatry.* **29** (1), 57–67.

Peddie, C. (2009). Rowanbank clinic embraces behavioural family therapy within the new forensic medium secure setting. *The Meriden Family Programme Newsletter.* 4–6.

Pekkala, E. & Merinder, L. (2002). *Psychoeducation for schizophrenia.* Cochrane Database Systematic Review. 2011 (6):CD002831. PMID: 12076455.

Pharoah, F., Mari, J., Rathbone, J. & Wong, W. (2010). *Family intervention for schizophrenia.* Cochrane Database Systematic Review. 2010 (12):CD000088. Published 2010 Dec 8. doi:10.1002/14651858.CD000088.pub2

Rapaport, J., Bellringer, S., Pinfold, V. & Huxley, P. (2007). Carers and confidentiality in mental healthcare: considering the role of the carer's assessment: a study of service users', informal carers' and practitioners' views. *Health and Social Care in the Community.* **14**, 357–65.

Richards, M., Doyle, M. & Cook, P. (2009). A literature review of family interventions for dual diagnosis: implications for forensic mental health services. *British Journal of Forensic Practice.* **11** (4), 39–49.

Ridley, J., McKeown, M., Machin, K., Rosengard, A., Little, S., Briggs, S., Jones, F. & Deypurkaystha, M. (2014). *Exploring family carer involvement in forensic mental health services.* Support in Mind Scotland, Edinburgh.

Robinson, L., Haskayne, D. & Larkin, M. (2017). How do carers view their relationship with forensic mental health services? *Journal of Forensic Psychology Research and Practice.* **17**, 232–48.

Ryan, T. (2002). Exploring the risk management strategies of informal carers of mental health service users. *Journal of Mental Health.* **11**, 17–25.

Savage, L. & McKeown, M. (1997). Towards a new model for practice in a HDU. *Psychiatric Care.* **4** (4), 182–86.

Seikkula, J. & Olson, M.E. (2003). The open dialogue approach to acute psychosis: Its poetics and micropolitics. *Family Process.* **42** (3), 403–18.

Simons, L., Petch, A. & Caplan, R. (2002). *'Don't they call it Seamless Care?': A Study of Acute Psychiatric Discharge.* Nuffield Centre for Community Care Studies/Scottish Executive Social Research.

Slade, M., Pinfold, V., Rapaport, J., Bellringer, S., Banerjee, S., Kuipers, E. & Huxley, P. (2007). Best practice when service users do not consent to sharing information with informal carers. *British Journal of Psychiatry.* **190**, 148–55.

Szmukler, G. & Holloway, F. (2001). 'Confidentiality in community psychiatry.' In: C. Cordess (ed.). *Confidentiality and Mental Health.* London: Jessica Kingsley, 53–67.

Tarrier, N., Haddock, G. & Barrowclough, C. (1998). 'Training and dissemination: research to practice in innovative psychosocial treatments for schizophrenia.' In: T. Wykes, N. Tarrier & S. Lewis (eds). *Outcome and Innovation in the Psychological Management of Schizophrenia.* Chichester: Wiley.

Tsang, H. (2002). Family needs and burdens of mentally ill offenders. *International Journal of Rehabilitation Research.* **25** (1), 25–32.

Vallentine, V., Tapp, J., Dudley, A., Wilson, C. & Moore, E. (2010). Psycho-educational group work for detained offender patients: understanding mental illness. *Journal of Forensic Psychiatry and Psychology.* **21**, 393–406.

Walker, H. (2004). Using psychosocial interventions within a high security hospital. *Nursing Times.* **100** (31), 36–39.

Walker, H., Connaughton, J., Wilson, I. & Martin, C. (2012). Improving outcomes for psychoses through the use of psycho-education; preliminary findings. *Journal of Psychiatric and Mental Health Nursing.* **19** (10), 881–90.

Walker, H., Trenoweth, S., Martin, C. & Ramm, M. (2013). Using repertory grid to establish patients' views of psycho-education. *Journal of Psychology and Psychotherapy.* **3**, 108.

Wallcraft, J., Amering, M., Freidin, J., Davar, B., Froggatt, D., Jafri, H., Javed, A., Katontoka, S., Raja, S., Rataemane, S., Steffen, S., Tyano, S., Underhill, C., Wahlberg, H., Warner, R. & Herrman, H. (2011). Partnerships for better mental health worldwide: WPA recommendations on best practice in working with service users and family informal carers. *World Psychiatry.* **10**, 229–36.

Worthington, A., Rooney, P. & Hannah, R. (2013). *The Triangle of Care. Carers Included: A Guide to Best Practice in Mental Healthcare in England.* 2nd edn. London: Carers Trust.

Chapter 8

Substance misuse, alcohol and working with families

Gemma Stacey-Emile

Introduction

This chapter will explore how important it is not only to work with individuals who misuse substances but also with their families. Treatment services have historically focused on the individual accessing help, and particularly on their motivation to engage with treatment. The National Institute for Health and Care Excellence (NICE 2007) promote a behaviour change flowchart which suggests that improvements should be made to service access to support those individuals who have difficulty with motivation. Each member of the family unit can have a significant impact on their loved one's recovery and engagement with services. Across the UK, there is an array of services for individuals and families who experience problems with substance misuse. Unfortunately, policies and interventions vary considerably according to locality.

Alcohol, drugs, prescribed and over-the-counter medication can all be misused, causing physical and psychological harm. According to the Department of Health (2018) and NICE (2015), alcohol is one of the largest avoidable risks for disease and death – excessive alcohol use has been linked to cancers of the mouth and breast, along with increased risk of developing dementia, disability and frailty. The current alcohol guidelines in the United Kingdom advise that men and women should drink no more than 14 units each week and should refrain from drinking if pregnant (NICE 2015). NICE (2018) provides clinical standards, quality standards and pathways for 'Alcohol use disorders' and 'Drug misuse' for individuals, family members and healthcare professionals regarding relevant treatment options.

There is evidence to suggest that, as well as working with individuals with substance misuse problems, working with their family, loved ones or 'concerned others' can have a very positive impact in terms of the individuals obtaining appropriate treatment (Harris 2018). It has also been suggested, by McCann *et al.* (2018), that the 'affected family member' can develop maladaptive coping mechanisms and may experience significant gaps in support and education.

Aims and learning outcomes

This chapter will offer an overview of the issues facing people who misuse alcohol and substances. Having completed the chapter, the reader will:

- Recognise key problems for the family where alcohol or substances are a problem
- Understand how working with a family focus can be helpful in these situations.

Substance misuse terminology and stigma

The *Diagnostic and Statistical Manual of Mental Disorders* (American Psychiatric Association 2013) recognises substance-related disorders resulting from the use of 10 separate classes of drugs and alcohol. There are two groups of substance-related disorders: substance use disorders and substance-induced disorders. The severity of the problem will be indicated by how many symptoms are identified. There are many self-assessment questionnaires available for the public to access, to help them determine if they are drinking too much, with further advice and tools to seek self-help or help from organisations.

Websites, such as Alcohol Change UK, Drinkaware and Drugwise, are free information sites that provide evidence-based information for the general public to access. The *Drug misuse and dependence: UK guidelines and clinical management* (Department of Health 2017) underpin various elements of substance misuse service practice, ensuring that individuals misusing any substances are offered evidence-based assessment and treatment. Within these guidelines, the impact of drug misuse on families and children is recognised, and there is a focus on collaborative working with partnership agencies to protect and improve the health and wellbeing of affected children. Treatment initiatives are also identified to improve the quality of life for family members. In the UK, the number of drug-related deaths due to overdose is the highest in Europe. In addition, people in treatment or in the criminal justice system who use opiates are six time more likely to die prematurely than people in the general population (Department of Health 2017).

Within healthcare services, it is important to consider the impact of terminology, as our choice of words can form prejudices and affect the way we care for individuals. This may be due to personal experience, what we have heard from colleagues, our attitudes, values and beliefs.

There are also legal aspects to consider in relation to substance use. It is essential to remember that some individuals may, over a lifetime, have periods of substance abuse without any significant issues affecting their day-to-day lives. However, the same individual may sometimes be under stress, for a variety of reasons (such as marriage break-up, loss of employment or childcare issues) and resort/relapse to past coping mechanises and 'misuse' their chosen substance once more, with more damaging effects.

Words and terminology can have a great impact on the individual. For instance, terms such as 'addict', 'alcoholic' and 'alcohol/drug abuser' can offer an unwelcome negative connotation, suggesting that individuals themselves are the 'problem'. Within the field of substance misuse, different approaches and philosophies may use words interchangeably and this must always be carefully considered. For example, Alcoholics Anonymous (2018) use the word 'alcoholic' and share their experiences to help others 'recover from alcoholism' by following a 12-step programme to make amends for past behaviour, while recognising that everyone has the ability to recover and lead a fulfilling life, free from alcohol.

Other organisations may use a Harm Reduction or Community Reinforcement Approach, which focuses on the individual's goals, whether this involves a reduction of substance use, total abstinence or a significant change in their associated behaviours such as safer injecting (Harris 2018, Barod 2018, SMART Recovery UK 2018). Organisations can provide a range of services for young people, family and friends, including group work, drop-ins, diversionary activities, complementary therapies, aftercare and brief interventions, but these will again vary depending on locality. General practitioners are often the first contact point for individuals and concerned family members but services and the involvement of primary care in drug treatment varies significantly (Department of Health 2017).

There continues to be a societal and cultural stigma surrounding mental health and substance misuse, which are often portrayed negatively by the media. Campaigns to reduce barriers and stigma in the workplace have been initiated by organisations such as Time to Change Wales (2017) and the World Health Organization. According to Alcohol Change (2018), reducing alcohol harm to individuals and society is difficult, due to the central role played by alcohol in many social interactions. There is a need to raise awareness of the harm caused by alcohol through knowledge and better policy and regulation. There is also a need to improve the nation's drinking behaviour and shift cultural norms, whilst providing better support and treatment.

Why do people misuse substances?

There are various reasons why individuals use and misuse substances, including over-the-counter medication and prescribed medication. These are listed in Table 8.1 on page 106.

The reasons why people drink alcohol and abuse substances vary a great deal, and it must be noted that the legal and illegal aspects of alcohol and drugs can significantly affect engagement and stigma. According to the Alcohol Health Alliance UK (2018), alcohol misuse can be linked to a range of social problems such as antisocial behaviour, domestic violence, ill health, violent crime, road traffic accidents and sexual assaults. There is also evidence suggesting that alcohol use is linked to child abuse and neglect: 37% of child deaths and serious injuries due to neglect are linked to parental drinking (Department of Health 2018).

Table 8.1: Positive and negative reasons for substance misuse

Positive reasons	Negative reasons
• Tastes nice	• I can't stop
• Helps me to relax	• Helps to block negative thoughts
• All my friends do it and it is sociable	• Helps me to sleep
• Gives me a bit of confidence	• I can't leave the house now without having a drink
• It is fun	• It has left me feeling scared
• It is legal	• It can be illegal
• Everyone else is doing it	• I feel under peer pressure to conform
• Blocks intrusive thoughts	• My physical health deteriorates

Overall there appears to be a functional gain for individuals drinking alcohol or using substances. For example, consuming alcohol may help block out feelings attributed to bereavement. Likewise, using drugs in a group of friends/peers, due to boredom and feelings of low self-worth, may replace negative feelings with more positive feelings, albeit in the short term and with potential longer-term negative effects. The context is an important factor to consider when discussing an individual's alcohol and substance use, as many people use alcohol and drugs as a coping mechanism to deal with negative feelings such as depression, stress, trauma and anxiety (Drugwise 2018, Alcohol Change 2018).

Effects of substance misuse on the person

It is important to recognise the internal and external barriers that people experience, and it is sometimes hard to accept that people are not ready to address these problems. For example, someone who has continued to misuse alcohol since their partner's death may not feel ready to experience the shock and numbness associated with grief (Alcohol Change 2018).

It is essential to recognise the physical and psychological factors involved in using and misusing substances, as this can be pivotal when individuals ask for help. Sometimes when loved ones are met with ultimatums within the family unit, the individual is 'forced' to make decisions to actively address their use. For example, a parent may not leave their child with their partner anymore because they know they are intoxicated and are concerned that they will not be able to look after the child appropriately.

These physical and psychological complexities can affect an individual's motivation to actively address and change their behaviour. The physical and psychological desire to carry on drinking can be difficult to address and motivating factors need to be considered in assessment sessions (Prochaska & DiClemente 1992). Substance use doesn't only affect the individual but also the whole family. Families are complex, and unique, so they require different approaches and services.

Firstly, all substance misuse services will perform an assessment, which focuses on a psychosocial and risk component. The assessment underpins the identification of treatment needs and the individual agrees their goal/s for treatment and recovery jointly with the assessor. The Self-Management and Recovery Training (UK) (SMART Recovery UK 2018) approach is often adopted by substance misuse services, the NHS, prisons and probation services within the UK. It aims to 'empower people with practical skills, tools and support so that they may manage their addictive behaviour and lead satisfying and meaningful lives.'

Within families where loved ones are misusing substances, there may often have been years of distrust, broken promises, tears, upset and arguments. This can often lead to relationship break-downs, financial concerns, housing issues, and employment/education disruptions. Family members invent their own ways of coping which can sometimes include colluding with the person, although the family members may not recognise this at the time. For instance, relatives will often pay off debts, limit money to access alcohol, buy alcohol/drugs, allow them to move back home/leave home in the hope that they can then control and influence their loved ones' often chaotic needs.

This behaviour can unfortunately escalate, leading to more specific problems for the families and carers. It is therefore important to identify the need to provide treatment for the substance misuse problem as well as the associated emotional and mental health issues. McCann *et al.* (2018) recognise that the harms identified through assessment of the individual misusing the substance are not limited to just the individual but can also affect family members. These 'harms' can have adverse implications for the family dynamics and for family members' wellbeing and willingness to carry out their supportive role. The stress of caring and living with individuals misusing substances can affect family members' employment, physical health and ability to maintain their own support networks.

Interventions that may be helpful for an individual

When there is a mental health and substance misuse problem, it is essential that all aspects of a person are explored, as this contributes to the wholeness and well-being of the individual (Working to Recovery 2016). Due to ongoing funding issues within healthcare around substance misuse services, services can be both statutory and non-statutory. Substance misuse teams are made up of nurses, doctors, recovery workers, social workers, occupational therapists, clinical psychologists, peer mentors, family therapists, counsellors and criminal justice services.

Within a psychosocial assessment, the following domains would be discussed, and problem areas highlighted, in order to assess the associated risks involved for both the individual and their family:

- Immediate risk
- Confirmation of substance misuse problem
- Degree of problem use or dependence
- Physical and mental health problems
- Social problems
- Family history
- Patient's understanding of treatment options and motivation for change
- Exploring the person's strengths
- Determining any need for substitute medication and other prescribing issues
- Assessing longer-term risks, including those associated with injecting
- Assessing parental responsibility if relevant (Department of Health 2018).

Treatment services are generally tiered, offering the least intrusive form of intervention first. For instance, a telephone triage system may be offered or an initial assessment so that the individual can be assessed and perhaps signposted to more specialist services, depending on the information provided. It would be normal for all these domains to be reviewed in line with the individual – a person-centred approach is generally taken to address the issues which are causing the main distress for the individual.

Within the assessment process, areas for further consideration may include:

- Physical dependence and withdrawal symptoms
- Physical complications such as blood-borne viruses, continued risky behaviour, liver disease, abscesses, overdose, sexual health problems and pregnancy
- Domestic violence, lack of social integration, abuse and risk of homelessness
- Child protection and safeguarding issues
- Impact of parents' physical and mental health on their parenting abilities
- Storage of illicit drugs, prescribed medication and drug paraphernalia.

Interventions that may be helpful for a family

As there are so many different services, charities and organisations offering support and advice for people affected by substance misuse, it is important that statutory services are aware of locally commissioned services that can support the family if there are concerns for children and affected family members. In the UK, organisations such as Adfam, Alcohol Change, Aquarius and Barnardo's provide specialist services to those who are affected by their loved one's substance misuse. These organisations all recognise the impact of substances used within the home and the associated behaviours.

Adfam have adopted the five-step method as an example of how to help family members in their own right (Orford *et al.* 2010). This approach is based on a theoretical appreciation of how family members can be affected by substance misuse, based on research evaluating what it is like to live with someone who misuses substances and then offering family members help in their own right. The way family members, children and young people cope with substance misuse within the family unit can manifest both physically and emotionally, as highlighted by McCann *et al.* (2018). When children and parents can discuss their feelings in a safe place, it reduces family-related harm from parental substance misuse (Templeton 2014). Action on Addiction (2018) in the UK has adopted the M-Pact (Moving parents and children together) programme, and the findings from Templeton (2014) suggest that this intervention offers improvements in children that include:

- School behaviour, engagement and attendance
- Dietary habits and physical hygiene
- Relationships, self-esteem and anxiety levels
- Reduced offending behaviour.

Benefits may also include:

- Reduction in parental substance misuse
- The removal of child protection plans/proceeding
- More family engagement with welfare and support services
- Improvements in family communication.

According to the Social Care Institute for Excellence (2011), the 'Think Family' agenda identifies risks, stressors and vulnerability factors increasing the likelihood of a poor outcome, as well as strengths, resources and protective factors that enable families to overcome adversity. Working with families is complex and, as previously mentioned, the context is key and the services need to meet the whole family. Unfortunately, this can be frustrating, as not all services are provided equitably throughout the UK. The Integrated Family Support Service provides a unique programme which the local authority can refer to if there are concerns about the welfare of children in relation to:

- Substance misuse
- Domestic violence/abuse

- History of violence or abusive behaviour
- Mental health issues.

The purpose of this service is to work with the whole family to help make positive changes and to reduce the risk of children being removed from the home (Children and Families (Wales) Measure, National Assembly for Wales, 2010).

Communication, skills and relationships

The skills required of the professionals across services are paramount for the engagement of individuals and family members. In *Drug misuse and dependence: UK guidelines and clinical management* (Department of Health 2017), the authors acknowledge the importance of building an effective therapeutic alliance with the individual, supported by collaboration, person-centred treatment and recovery care planning. It is also recognised that the professional needs to utilise their motivation and their clinical and planning skills to facilitate the process of treatment and recovery.

Offering a humanistic approach, based on the principles described by Rogers (1961) and Egan (2013), allows individuals to feel empowered and able to make choices in relation to their problems. The underlying philosophies are based on individual motivation, recognising that each person is unique, with their own individual sense of achievement. The relationship between the professional and the person and family is central in creating a positive view of their needs and offering hope and compassion, with realistic opportunities emerging and being offered. Enabling the individual and family to feel comfortable about engaging with services and treatment is key.

Working with people within healthcare structures requires clear, effective communication. Confidence, self-awareness and emotional intelligence are also important factors when trying to engage people in treatment services. A sharing of knowledge and experience can alleviate fears and anxiety in others, and create a comfortable environment that is both welcoming and non-threatening. The circular transactional model of communication, based on Bateson (cited in McCabe & Timmins 2013), offers a link to the broader aspects of communication and identifies intrinsic and extrinsic factors.

Within the nurse/assessor–individual relationship, successful communication can be achieved through discussion, feedback and validation (McCabe & Timmins 2013). Individuals often only communicate what they think others will understand, and feelings of embarrassment, helplessness and ignorance may cloud the communication process so that a false picture of the situation is being shared. In time, and once a good/therapeutic relationship has been achieved, the individual may feel able to share their thoughts honestly, recognising that the practitioner can help and/or facilitate change/acceptance. Working with people who misuse substances requires patience, commitment, and deep understanding regarding the complexities of the substances and their biological and psychological effects. Engaging with all the family members enables the healthcare professional to reinforce the fact that the individual does still have control and power over their own choices (SMART Recovery UK 2018, Department of Health 2017).

The transtheoretical model of change (Prochaska & DiClemente 1999) offers a clear structure and framework for policy makers, service providers, clinicians and mental health practitioners to outline specific behaviours that individuals want to change. It is best to use this model, along with the SMART Recovery Model (2018), with a non-judgemental attitude whilst building a therapeutic relationship that provides a clear supportive focus. Motivational interviewing, dialectical behaviour therapy, group work and trialogue can influence how well individuals engage with services, and there is strong conceptual and empirical evidence for the benefits offered by these interventions (Amering et al. 2012, Cooper 2011). There is evidence to suggest that working within trialogues (carers, friends and mental health workers) can enable change for all those involved with loved ones and family members (Amering et al. 2012). The inclusion of all those involved within the family is clearly vital for recovery-orientated mental health practice and research (Amering and Schmolke 2009).

To summarise, due to the complexities of individual substance misuse and the effects it can have on all members of the family, it is important that help is sought for *all* those affected, as there may be both short- and long-term effects on physical health and wellbeing for everyone. There are some very useful UK websites, but consideration must be given to what is available locally. Healthcare practitioners need good core communication skills to enable people to access the right treatment at the right time. Having access to a range of services is key to enabling the family to address their problems and minimise poor functioning and inability to cope.

Illustrative case study

Fiona and Paul have been married for 15 years and they have two children, Sara aged 7 and Luke aged 13. They both work and have parents living nearby who are supportive and look after the children occasionally after school. Paul has a history of using alcohol excessively and he currently links this to his job. He is drinking excessively and he has missed some days of work, due to being too hungover to go in. This has caused upset. Fiona's parents have always thought Paul drinks too much anyway, leaving Fiona to look after the whole family and work full-time as well. At family gatherings, Paul has always had a tendency to drink and become rowdy and has upset some family members in the past by making unwelcome comments.

This time Fiona has had enough and thinks that the children are being affected by his drinking, as they see him drink regularly and they have found him asleep on the sofa in the morning after a heavy drinking session. She has told him to go and get help and has said she will move out until he does.

Outcome:

Fiona has not contacted alcohol services before and doesn't know where to start. When she looks on the internet, she is left confused about who to contact and is now debating whether to contact anyone at all as it seems too confusing. A few days later, after another argument about Paul's drinking, she phones some of the numbers she found. They all say that, unless her husband calls himself, they cannot offer to arrange an appointment for him. She tells Paul this. He refuses to make an appointment and says he will sort himself out.

Paul's drinking escalates, as he has been given a verbal warning about being late for work. Fiona contacts some of the alcohol service numbers again – pleading with them and saying that her husband has a problem and needs help. They reiterate that they cannot offer him an appointment but they say that she could have a carer's assessment appointment and that this would be confidential, where she would have the option to talk to an alcohol worker about how she is feeling and coping.

Reflection

- List three key points to consider when working with someone using substances as a coping mechanism.
- List five reasons why someone may be using substances.
- Why is it important to consider the whole family when working with individuals? List three areas for consideration.

Conclusion

It is essential to offer help and support when working with people who are misusing substances and evidence suggests that the impact of substance misuse is significant for all family members. Substance misuse, especially alcohol, causes avoidable physical and emotional harm. It is therefore important to offer the right help and signpost individuals to services as soon as a problem arises. Service availability differs across the UK and also depends on the severity of substance misuse, which must be assessed and considered.

References

Action on Addiction (2018). *Annual Review*. https://www.actiononaddiction.org.uk/about/about-us/our-reports-and-publications (last accessed 30.9.2019).

Alcohol Change (2018). https://alcoholchange.org.uk/ (last accessed 29.8.2019).

Alcoholics Anonymous (2018). https://www.alcoholics-anonymous.org.uk/ (last accessed 29.8.2019).

Alcohol Health Alliance UK (2018). http://ahauk.org/ (last accessed 29.8.2019).

American Psychiatric Association (2013). *Diagnostic and Statistical Manual of Mental Disorders*. 5th edn. Washington DC.

Amering, M., Mikus, M. & Steffen, S. (2012). Recovery in Austria: Mental health trialogue. *International Review of Psychiatry*. **24** (1), 11–18.

Amering, M. & Schmolke, M. (2009). *Recovery in Mental Health: Reshaping Scientific and Clinical Responsibilities*. London: Wiley.

Barod (2018). http://barod.cymru/what-we-do/services-we-provide/ (last accessed 29.8.2019).

Cooper, B.D. (ed.) (2011). *Developing Services in Mental Health-Substance Use*. Oxford: Radcliffe Publishing.

Drugwise (2018). https://www.drugwise.org.uk/ (last accessed 29.8.2019).

Department of Health (2017). *Drug misuse and dependence: UK guidelines and clinical management*. https://assets.publishing.service.gov.uk/government/uploads/system/uploads/attachment_data/file/673978/clinical_guidelines_2017.pdf (last accessed 29.8.2019).

Department of Health (2018). *Statistics from the NI Substance Misuse database 2016/17*. https://www.health-ni.gov.uk/news/statistics-ni-substance-misuse-database-201617 (last accessed 29.8.2019).

Egan, G. (2013). *The Skilled Helper: A Problem-Management and Opportunity-Development Approach to Helping, International*. 10th edn. UK: Brooks Cole Cengage Learning.

Harris, P. (2018). *Developing Effective Services for Adolescents, Families & Adults*. https://www.philharris.online/alcohol (last accessed 29.8.2019).

McCabe, C. & Timmins, F. (2013). *Communication Skills for Nursing Practice*. 2nd edn. Basingstoke: Palgrave Macmillan.

McCann, T.V., Stephenson, J. & Lubman, D.I. (2018). Affected family member coping with a relative with alcohol and/or other drug misuse: A cross sectional survey questionnaire. *International Journal of Mental Health Nursing*. **23** (3), 687–96.

National Assembly for Wales (2010). *Children and Families (Wales) Measure*, Cardiff, National Assembly for Wales http://www.legislation.gov.uk/mwa/2010/1/contents (last accessed 30.9.2019).

National Institute for Health and Care Excellence (NICE) (2007). *Drug misuse in over 16s: psychosocial interventions*. London: NICE.

National Institute for Health and Care Excellence (NICE) (2011). *Alcohol-use disorders: assessment and management of harmful drinking and alcohol dependence*. London: NICE.

National Institute for Health and Care Excellence (NICE) (2015). *Dementia, disability and frailty in later life – mid-life approaches to delay or prevent onset*. https://www.nice.org.uk/guidance/ng16/chapter/1-Recommendations (last accessed 29.8.2019).

National Institute for Health and Care Excellence (NICE) (2018). *Alcohol-use disorders overview*. London: NICE.

Orford, J., Copello, A., Velleman, R. & Templeton, L. (2010). Family members affected by a close relative's addiction: the stress-strain-coping-support model. *Drugs: Education, Prevention and Policy*. **17** (s1), 36–43.

Prochaska, J.O. & DiClemente, C.C. (1992). Stages of change in the modification of problem behaviors. *Progress in Behavior Modification*. **28**, 183–218.

Prochaska, J.O. & DiClemente, C.C. (1999). 'Toward a comprehensive transtheoretical model of change: Stages of change and addictive behaviors' In: W.R. Miller & N. Health (eds). *Treating Addictive Behaviors*. 2nd edition. New York and London: Plenum Press.

Rogers, C. (1961). *On Becoming a Person: A Therapist's View of Psychotherapy*. London: Constable.

Smart Recovery UK. https://smartrecovery.org.uk/ (last accessed 29.8.2019).

Social Care Institute for Excellence (2011). The Family Model (The Model), cited in the 'Think Child, Think Parent, Think Family' guidance. https://www.scie.org.uk/publications/guides/guide30/introduction/thinkchild.asp (last accessed 29.8.2019).

Templeton, L. (2014). Supporting families living with parental substance misuse: the M-PACT (Moving Parents and Children Together) Programme Child and Family. *Social Work*. **19**, 76–88.

Time to Change Wales (2017). http://www.timetochangewales.org.uk/en/ (last accessed 29.8.2019).

Working to Recovery (2016). http://www.workingtorecovery.co.uk/ (last accessed 29.8.2019).

Chapter 9

Working with military veterans

Clare Crole-Rees, Neil Kitchiner, Dean Whybrow

Introduction

This chapter focuses on working with veterans from the UK armed forces. The aim is to offer the reader an insight into the particular challenges that face veterans and their families and a skills-based example of how to support veterans in their recovery from military-related post-traumatic stress disorder (PTSD) by involving their families. To achieve this aim, we define what is meant by the term 'veteran', describe the type of support available to serving military personnel and veterans, and discuss the impact of mental health problems on veterans' families, before introducing cognitive behavioural conjoint therapy via an illustrative case study.

We would like to thank our colleagues at Anglia Ruskin University for help with an earlier draft of this chapter.

Aims and learning outcomes

The aim of this chapter is to explore the needs of families of veterans and consider ways in which mental health practitioners can be helpful. Having completed this chapter, the reader will have:

- An understanding of the mental health needs of veterans
- An appreciation of one evidence-based model that might be helpful to use with families.

Defining veterans

The term 'veteran' can be defined as 'somebody who has extensive experience in a particular field' (Soanes & Stevenson 2009). Internationally, there are different understandings of the term and what it actually means within an armed forces context. Historically, it might mean 'service personnel with combat experience' (Havighurst, Eaton, Baughman & Burgess 1951). More recently, it has been used to describe military personnel leaving the forces after very different lengths of service or military experience (Dandeker, Wessely, Iversen & Ross 2006). The UK government adopts an inclusive approach to defining a veteran, whereas other nations might exclude people who have not deployed on operations. Dandeker *et al.* (2006) suggest that the strength of an inclusive definition incorporating everybody (even new recruits with one day's service) is that it protects early service leavers. This may be important because early service leavers have been identified as a group that are more vulnerable to difficulties when transitioning to civilian life (Bergman, Burdett & Greenberg 2014) and to experiencing mental health issues (Buckman *et al.* 2013).

Finally, just because somebody qualifies for the label of 'veteran', it does not mean that they will necessarily identify with it, even after several years' service and combat experience (Burdett *et al.* 2012). Within a UK military setting, the term 'veteran' includes everyone who has been associated with the armed forces, regardless of experience or length of service. This definition also means that the families of veterans will include people whose partners come from the entire spectrum of ex-service personnel (i.e. a heterogeneous population).

Mental health service provision for military personnel and veterans

The armed forces depend on their personnel to achieve the objectives set by the government of the day. Whilst it is true that technology plays an increasingly important role in delivering an effective fighting force, human beings are still required – and the military would not be fit for purpose without them (Boot 2015). It is important that these personnel are trained in their military roles, whether they are infantry, engineers, aircrew, medics, sailors or chefs. The military goes to great lengths to achieve this by ensuring a minimum standard of basic training as well as role-specific training and further specialist training throughout a service person's career. In addition, the military provides food, clothing and shelter, all of which may help improve morale and promote resiliency – indeed, improved nutrition in the developed world has been considered an important factor in promoting health (McKeown 1991). In addition, the armed forces have a substantial medical service, including a mental health service, designed to optimise health and wellbeing for military personnel.

It could be argued that military personnel are a self-selecting group of fit young people interested in military life and also a group in which people are filtered out early in the application process if they are not suited to the environment. However, this does not explain why military personnel seem to report more symptoms of mental ill health than the civilian working population (Goodwin *et al.* 2015). When making this comparison, these latter authors describe a rate of common mental disorder in the general population of 8.4% in males and 12% in females. By comparison they report a military rate of psychiatric disorder of 18% in males and 25.6% in females.

In spite of this, most service personnel seem to do well when they leave the forces. Those personnel who leave early (within four years) are more vulnerable to mental health problems than those who have completed their full term of service (Buckman *et al.* 2013). This may be because there are higher rates of childhood adversity and pre-existing mental health problems in early service leavers (Buckman *et al.* 2012).

Reservists are also more vulnerable to common mental health problems, particularly PTSD and alcohol misuse, than regular serving personnel. Research has shown that increased rates of PTSD in reservists were strongly associated with problems at home, both during and after deployment, and a perceived lack of support from the military (Harvey *et al.* 2011). It therefore appears that, although military populations may on the whole be resilient when transitioning to veteran life, specific groups experience vulnerability to mental health difficulties during service and for some this may continue or develop once they leave the service.

To better support those individuals in service, the armed forces have a comprehensive medical organisation that provides both primary and secondary care services. This includes a mental health service consisting of psychiatrists, community mental health nurses, clinical nurse specialists, social workers and psychologists. Access to military mental health services is via GP referral, although self-referral has recently been tested to good effect (Kennedy *et al.* 2016) and may be introduced more widely at some future stage. In addition, psychological resilience following a potentially traumatic event is promoted via the peer support system Trauma Risk Management, which promotes timely access to care for those in need (Whybrow, Jones & Greenberg 2015). When accessing the mental health service, military personnel can be reassured that it seems to be an effective service, with a high recovery rate reported by a military community mental health team, when compared to equivalent civilian services – 68% recovery rate in the military, compared to 52% in the equivalent National Health Service (Clark, Layard & Smithies 2008, Gould *et al.* 2008).

The mental health service provision is focused on supporting serving personnel. In addition, there are some situations, such as foreign deployments, where family members may also be able to access military healthcare. Military personnel have access to an occupationally focused, comprehensive and effective mental health service that forms part of a wider medical service and is well integrated with the armed forces. This does not mean that it is a perfect service or that everybody recovers; indeed, a number of people will be medically discharged with mental health problems each year. For example, from April 2011 to March 2016, it was reported that 15% (n = 1,236) of army medical discharges were for mental health problems (MOD 2016a) and mental ill health was the second highest reason for medical discharge from the armed forces (Diehle & Greenberg 2015). Other individuals may also go on to present with service-related mental health problems as civilians (van Hoorn *et al.* 2013).

Military mental health services remain available to veterans for the first six months following discharge and during the early stages of the transition to civilian life (Murrison 2010). Following this, veterans have access to a number of sources of support, from the NHS and veteran charities. Although the military has a range of strategies to support those in need, a more joined-up approach is recommended for supporting those service leavers who may find it difficult to access help (Nottingham & Bunn 2016). Sources of support for veterans include a government-run veterans' helpline, third sector organisations, veterans-focused services and an online service for those experiencing psychological distress (Murrison 2010).

Veterans' mental health

The prevalence of mental disorders amongst UK veterans' populations has been estimated to be 10.2% amongst regular veterans and 10.9% for reservist veterans (Diehle & Greenberg, 2015). The most prevalent disorders are depression (20%), alcohol misuse and anxiety (Iversen & Greenberg 2009). Research shows that some groups are more vulnerable to mental disorders, such as those with physical health problems (Stevelink *et al.* 2014) and early service leavers (Bergman *et al.* 2014). Post-traumatic stress disorder (PTSD) remains a rarer problem, which affects approximately 4% of veterans (Fear *et al.* 2010). In comparison to the civilian population, it would seem that military personnel are more likely to report symptoms consistent with common mental health problems. Offering timely care is likely to improve the mental health of those veterans who are suffering ongoing problems (Kitchiner *et al.* 2012).

Impact on families

Little is known about the impact of deployment on partner relationships among UK military personnel. Rowe *et al.* (2013) have found that risk factors for negative relationship change following deployment to Iraq include the presence of PTSD and other common mental health problems. They argue that these individuals are at risk of suffering relationship breakdown and may benefit from intervention. This follows previous research in the US which also found that deployment to a hostile war zone was associated with increased relationship problems (Meis *et al.* 2010). Recent US studies of personnel deployed to Afghanistan and Iraq have looked at family functioning post-deployment: 75% reported at least one family adjustment issue, and 54% reported at least one incidence of verbal or physical abuse towards their partner (Sayers *et al.* 2009).

It is clear that the mental health of returning service personnel affects children's well-being, as well as family functioning and relationship satisfaction. It is therefore important that the needs of the entire family are considered by mental health service providers. In a US study of veterans receiving treatment for PTSD, nearly 80% were interested in greater family involvement in their care (Batten *et al.* 2009).

In the UK, various projects have been set up to support the partners and children of veterans, and there is an increasing awareness of their importance. For example, in Wales, The Listen In service (Mottershed *et al.* 2016) was created to provide a comprehensive resource to support families and carers in helping veterans gain sustained recovery from issues brought about through military action (such as substance misuse and psychosocial problems including PTSD), and help them rebuild normal productive lives. Listen In was also set up to help family members and carers deal with their own issues and life challenges, brought about through caring for veterans (Mottershead, Bray & Ellahi 2016).

The National Institute for Clinical Excellence (NICE) recommends couples therapy for a range of different disorders, including alcohol dependence (see Chapter 8) and depression. It also recognises the value of including families, to support people with PTSD, although there is no clear evidence base to support this as yet (NICE 2005). However, there is a developing body of research from the US and the UK suggesting that couples therapy for PTSD is effective (Monson, Fredman, *et al.* 2012). This is consistent with evidence suggesting the importance of involving the family and partner when working with veterans with PTSD. The next section offers a case study describing how a veteran with PTSD and his wife were treated with a couples-based therapy, Cognitive Behavioural Conjoint Therapy.

Cognitive Behavioural Conjoint Therapy (CBCT)

'CBCT (Cognitive-Behavioral Conjoint Therapy) for PTSD is a time-limited, manualised, disorder-specific conjoint therapy with the simultaneous goals of improving PTSD and enhancing intimate relationship functioning' (Monson, Fredman, *et al.* 2012, p. 4). Research has demonstrated that there is a strong association between a diagnosis of PTSD in veterans and relationship difficulties (Kessler, Walters & Forthofer 1998). Evidence also suggests that the health of intimate relationships is a factor in treatment engagement (Meis *et al.* 2010). More specifically, the involvement of partners in trauma-focused out-patient therapy reduces drop-out rates and improves adherence to the interventions (Monson, Fredman, *et al.* 2012).

Well-meaning partners often functionally collude with their loved one's emotional, cognitive and behavioural avoidance, which maintains their PTSD (Ehlers & Clark 2000). This in turn reduces feelings of closeness, intimacy and relationship satisfaction. Many veterans have difficulties in labelling and expressing emotions. Stigma related to mental distress increases emotional avoidance, levels of anger and aggression, and there is a particular association between emotional numbing and low relationship satisfaction. Emotional numbing symptoms are less responsive to existing individual evidence-based therapies for PTSD (Asmundson, Stapleton & Taylor 2004).

The individual's negative appraisals about the traumatic event, its sequelae and their own symptoms are a primary barrier to their recovery from PTSD (Ehlers & Clark 2000). These appraisals, or 'stuck points', contribute to emotional and cognitive avoidance of the trauma memory, which prevents processing and also leads to maladaptive coping behaviours such as excessive drinking or hypervigilance.

CBCT addresses the interacting behavioural, cognitive and emotional processes involved in PTSD and its associated relationship problems. It addresses specific avoidance behaviours that may prevent new learning and reduction in emotional distress. Emotional processes that maintain PTSD (such as numbing, avoidance of expression and high levels of hostility and anger) are targeted through psycho-education about emotions, a dyadic intervention strategy to reduce expressed anger and hostility, and communication skills training to improve intimate relationship satisfaction. Cognitive mechanisms that maintain PTSD are also targeted by using the individual's partner to facilitate processing of these misappraisals and to generate a new meaning for the trauma.

Monson and Fredman (2012) found that CBCT resulted in clinically significant reduction in PTSD severity and improvement in relationship satisfaction when compared to a waiting list control. The following case study describes a patient who was treated successfully by a veterans' service in Wales, and highlights how CBCT can be applied in clinical practice with veterans.

Illustrative case study of Cognitive Behavioural Conjoint Therapy (CBCT)

Background information

Dave and Liz were a married couple in their late 50s with three adult children and two young grandchildren. Dave was an army veteran and served 22 years, during which time he was deployed to a number of combat environments. He presented with a long history of recurrent depressive episodes and delayed-onset PTSD, triggered by news reports of atrocities in Syria, particularly images showing children killed by bombs.

Dave was assessed individually before meeting jointly with his partner. During this session, we obtained information about his personal and service history and his current circumstances. A full assessment of his PTSD symptoms, nature of the traumatic memories and precipitating factors was obtained. In common with many ex-servicemen he had experienced multiple and cumulative traumatic events that contributed to the development of his PTSD. He described difficulties with emotional and physical intimacy in his relationship and avoided showing Liz when he was upset. He tended to avoid crowded places, such as shops and restaurants, and avoided reminders of his army career. Negative appraisals included a belief that he was to blame for a child getting killed in Oman, that he himself was 'broken' because of his symptoms, and that if Liz knew how he was feeling then she would leave him.

We opted to target his symptoms using CBCT. We felt that this would be an effective treatment as we could target specific appraisals rather than re-living a number of multiple and cumulative events. In addition, CBCT would target his chronic cognitive, emotional and behavioural avoidance, and could also address his explicit goal of improving his relationship satisfaction.

Treatment overview
Phase 1: Rationale for treatment, and education about PTSD and relationships
Phase 1 focuses on psycho-education regarding PTSD and the CBCT therapy. We explored the cycle of PTSD symptoms and discussed how treatment would use their relationship to decrease Dave's avoidance and emotional numbing and consider new ways of seeing the event, himself and others.

Phase 1 also focuses on identifying and reducing negative and hostile behaviours within the relationship. Strategies for reducing negative affect and anger, such as time-out, slowed breathing, and simple communication techniques, are introduced. Dave and Liz both completed a self-report questionnaire (Trauma Impact Questionnaire), in order to help them understand how the traumatic events had affected them across different cognitive domains.

Phase 2: Satisfaction enhancement and undermining avoidance
Phase 2 focuses on developing skills to improve communication between the couple and overcoming avoidance within a relationship. It introduces listening skills as a way of slowing down and improving communication, before developing skills in identifying and sharing a range of feelings, both 'positive' and 'negative'. These techniques helped to reduce Dave's symptoms of numbing and emotional avoidance.

We then worked on identifying and sharing thoughts in order to improve understanding of themselves and their partner, and to introduce the idea that their perceptions of events influence their emotional responses. The UNSTUCK process, which is the core cognitive intervention within the CBCT model, was introduced. We identified an upsetting thought that had come up during Dave's homework assignment – 'If I express my feelings then Liz will think I am weak'. We then together brainstormed and tested a range of alternative perspectives on this to develop the new, balanced thought 'Liz feels closer to me when I share my feelings'. Finally, in this phase we introduced problem-solving techniques to help the couple develop a range of solutions to identified problems within the relationship.

Phase 3: Making meaning of the trauma and end of therapy
In Phase 3, processing of the traumatic events takes place through identifying and working on maladaptive appraisals or 'stuck points' about the events, their causes and their impact, using the UNSTUCK process. These stuck points are seen as barriers to acceptance of the traumatic events. As alternative more realistic appraisals are generated, the couple moves to a fully contextualised and elaborated view, in which adaptive information is incorporated. We started by working with barriers to acceptance of the worst traumatic event, which for Dave was 'If I accept that it happened then I am betraying the victims'. In the remaining sessions, we worked on stuck points within the cognitive domains of blame ('It was my fault'), trust ('People are capable of terrible things and therefore no-one should be trusted'), control ('If I express my emotions I will lose control and have a breakdown') and emotional and physical closeness ('I must keep Liz at arm's length in order to protect her from my PTSD') before identifying and addressing stuck points that had interfered with post-traumatic growth.

Therapy outcome
At the end of therapy and at six-month follow-up, Dave no longer met diagnostic criteria for PTSD or depression. Both Dave and Liz reported a significant improvement in their relationship satisfaction, including sexual satisfaction. He demonstrated a marked improvement in his emotional expression, which enabled effective processing of distressing memories and experiences and enhanced intimacy within the relationship.

Collaborative behavioural tasks systematically exposed Dave to feared situations and reminders. He reported that his anxiety in response to these situations had gradually reduced until he was able to go to crowded restaurants and to cinemas with Liz. This in turn facilitated new learning that these situations were safe and that he was not under current threat. Dave reported that Liz's help in reframing painful appraisals related to the traumatic experiences and their aftermath was invaluable in allowing him to accept the reality of these experiences. In particular, his maintaining beliefs ('I am broken' and 'If I show Liz how I am feeling then she will leave me') were reframed and updated, and his accompanying feelings of shame dissipated. Overall both Dave and Liz reported high levels of satisfaction with the treatment and a significant reduction in pre- and post-therapy clinical measures.

Reflection
- What might be the main considerations for you when working with a veteran, before inviting family members to join a treatment plan?

Conclusion
Military veterans living with mental health problems are considered to be a unique group by the UK government due to their complex biopsychosocial needs. The term

'veteran' means different things to different people, with some arguing for a tighter definition to exclude veterans who have not completed basic training or deployed to a war zone. Here in the UK we have adopted an inclusive approach to the term, offering support to all veterans, from those who have served one day to those who have completed a full career.

A comprehensive and effective mental health service exists for serving members of the UK armed forces. However, not everybody recovers to the point that they are able to continue serving, and mental health problems are the second-highest reason for medical discharge. Although the majority of service personnel experience a positive transition into civilian life, for an important minority this transition may be more difficult, particularly when it includes living with service-related mental health problems. Research studies have demonstrated that military personnel report more symptoms of common mental health problems than their civilian counterparts. Indeed, it is estimated that 10% of veterans will experience a mental health problem. It is therefore clear that supporting this occupational group should be seen as a priority area for the military and NHS health services to invest in.

In addition, research increasingly suggests that the mental health of veterans, particularly following deployments, has an impact on the mental health and wellbeing of their partners and children, and that relationship functioning and satisfaction is negatively impacted by their mental health issues. Therefore, there is an increasing awareness of the importance of family interventions both in treating the mental health of the veteran and in improving relationship satisfaction and preventing relationship breakdown.

The UK military and the government have taken steps to support military personnel and their families as they transition from military to civilian life. However, a clear, integrated model of care for veterans and their families, with a single point of access, is still lacking. This issue is compounded because care and support is offered by a range of different organisations, including the military, the NHS and the third sector. Whilst a single point of access may be helpful, there are potential benefits offered by specialist veteran-focused services able to deliver novel and evidence-based interventions to support veterans who often have a range of complex needs.

There is a need for further research into how best to encourage veterans to seek help for mental health problems (both whilst serving and as veterans) from NHS services and charities. Research shows that involvement of significant others is one way to facilitate engagement and improve outcomes. We have therefore described how Conjoint Cognitive Behavioural Therapy might be one approach to helping veterans with PTSD, by recruiting family members or significant others to become co-therapists to support the veteran in their recovery from military-related PTSD.

Finally, increased awareness of the expertise that is available in veteran-focused NHS services may enable clinicians to more effectively signpost those in need to an early psychological intervention. After all, it is not only service users who may find the current array of services for veterans confusing to navigate, though the UK armed forces do provide some information about this for veterans during the discharge process. In addition to veteran-focused NHS services, and information available via military (MOD 2016b) and NHS (NHS England 2015) websites, clinicians may also wish to consider signposting to third sector organisations who may be well placed to support veterans and their families as they navigate a care pathway that enables them to access the right treatment at the right time and in the right place so that services are a positive resource on their journey of recovery.

References

Asmundson, G.J., Stapleton, J. & Taylor, S. (2004). Are avoidance and numbing distinct PTSD symptom clusters? *Journal of Traumatic Stress*. **17**, 467–75.

Batten, S., Drapalski, A.L., Decker, M.L., DeViva, J.C., Morris, L. J., Mann M.A. & Dixon, L.B. (2009). Veteran interest in family involvement in PTSD treatment. *Psychological Services*. **6** (3), 184–89.

Bergman, B.P., Burdett, H.J. & Greenberg, N. (2014). Service life and beyond – institution or culture? *The RUSI Journal*. **159** (5), 60–68. http://doi.org/10.1080/03071847.2014.969946 (last accessed 30.8.2019).

Boot, M. (2015). There is still nothing smarter than boots on the ground. https://www.newsweek.com/there-still-nothing-smarter-boots-ground-347336 (last accessed 30.8.2019).

Buckman, J.E.J., Forbes, H.J., Clayton, T., Jones, M., Jones, N., Greenberg, N., *et al*. (2013). Early Service leavers: a study of the factors associated with premature separation from the UK Armed Forces and the mental health of those that leave early. *European Journal of Public Health*. **23** (3), 410–415.

Burdett, H., Woodhead, C., Iversen, A.C., Wessely, S., Dandeker, C., & Fear, N. T. (2012). 'Are you a veteran?' Understanding of the term 'veteran' among UK ex-Service personnel: a research note. *Armed Forces & Society*. **39** (4), 751–59. http://doi.org/10.1177/0095327x12452033 (last accessed 30.8.2019).

Clark, D., Layard, R. & Smithies, R. (2008). *Improving Access to Psychological Therapy: Initial Evaluation of the Two Demonstration Sites*. London: London School for Economic Performance.

Dandeker, C., Wessely, S., Iversen, A. & Ross, J. (2006). What's in a name? Defining and caring for 'veterans': The United Kingdom in international perspective. *Armed Forces & Society*. **32** (2), 161–77. http://doi.org/10.1177/0095327x05279177 (last accessed 30.8.2019).

Diehle, J. & Greenberg, N. (2015). *Counting the Costs*. London: Help for Heroes; King's Centre for Military Health Research. https://www.kcl.ac.uk/kcmhr/publications/assetfiles/2015/Diehle2015.pdf (last accessed 30.8.2019).

Ehlers, A. & Clark, D. (2000). A cognitive model of post-traumatic stress disorder. *Behaviour Research and Therapy*. **38** (4), 319–45.

Fear, N., Jones, M., Murphy, D., Hull, L., Iversen, A.C., Coker, B., *et al*. (2010). What are the consequences of deployment to Iraq and Afghanistan on the mental health of the UK armed forces? A cohort study. *The Lancet*. **375** (9728), 1783–97.

Goodwin, L., Wessely, S., Hotopf, M., Jones, M., Greenberg, N., Rona, R.J., Hull, L. & Fear, N.T. (2015). Are common mental disorders more prevalent in the UK serving military compared to the general working population? *Psychological Medicine: A Journal of Research in Psychiatry and the Allied Sciences*. **45** (09), 1881–91. http://doi.org/10.1017/S0033291714002980 (last accessed 30.8.2019).

Gould, M., Sharpley, J. & Greenberg, N. (2008). Patient characteristics and clinical activities at a British military department of community mental health. *Psychiatric Bulletin*. **32** (3), 99–102. http://doi.org/10.1192/pb.bp.107.016337 (last accessed 30.8.2019).

Harvey, S.B., Hatch, S.L., Jones, M., Hull, L., Jones, N., Greenberg, N., Dandeker, C., Fear, N. & Wessley, S. (2011). Coming home: Social functioning and the mental health of UK reservists on return from deployment to Iraq or Afghanistan. *Annals of Epidemiology*. **23** (9), 666–72.

Havighurst, R.J., Eaton, W.H., Baughman, J.W. & Burgess, E. W. (1951). *The American Veteran Back Home; a Study of Veteran Readjustment*. Oxford: Longmans, Green.

Iversen, A.C. & Greenberg, N. (2009). Mental health of regular and reserve military veterans. *Advances in Psychiatric Treatment*. **15** (2), 100–106. http://doi.org/10.1192/apt.bp.107.004713 (last accessed 30.8.2019).

Iversen, A., van Staden, L. & Hacker Hughes, J. (2009). The prevalence of common mental disorders and PTSD in the UK military: using data from a clinical interview based study. *BMC Psychiatry*. **9**, 68.

Kennedy, I., Whybrow, D., Jones, N., Sharpley, J. & Greenberg, N. (2016). A service evaluation of self-referral to military mental health teams. *Occupational Medicine*. **66** (5), 394–98. http://doi.org/10.1093/occmed/kqw044 (last accessed 30.8.2019).

Kessler, R.C., Walters, E. & Forthofer, M. (1998). The social consequences of psychiatric disorders: 3. Probability of marital stability. *American Journal of Psychiatry.* **155**, 1092–96.

Kitchiner, N.J., & Bisson, J.I. (2015). Phase I Development of an optimal integrated care pathway for veterans discharged from the armed forces. *Military Medicine.* **180** (7), 766–73.

Kitchiner, N.J., Roberts, N.P., Wilcox, D. & Bisson, J.I. (2012). Systematic review and meta-analyses of psychosocial interventions for veterans of the military. *European Journal of Psychotraumatology.* **3** (2012) Incl Supplements.

McKeown, T. (1991). *The Origins of Human Disease.* Chichester: Wiley Blackwell.

Meis, L.A., Barry, R., Kehle, S., Erbes, C.R. & Polusny, M.A. (2010). Relationship adjustment, PTSD symptoms and treatment utilization among coupled National Guard soldiers deployed to Iraq. *Journal of Family Psychology.* **24**, 560–67.

Ministry of Defence (MOD) (2016a). *Annual Medical Discharges in the UK Regular Armed Forces 1 April 2011 – 31 March 2016.* London: MOD.

Ministry of Defence (MOD) (2016b). *Veterans UK.* https://www.gov.uk/government/organisations/veterans-uk (last accessed 30.8.2019).

Monson, C. & Fredman, S. (2012). *Cognitive-Behavioral Conjoint Therapy for PTSD: harnessing the healing power of relationships.* New York: Guildford Press.

Monson, C., Fredman, S., Macdonald, A., Pukay-Martin, N., Resick, P. & Schnurr, P.P. (2012). Effect of cognitive-behavioral couple therapy for PTSD: a randomized controlled trial. *Journal of the American Medical Association.* **308** (7), 700–709.

Mottershead, R., Bray, B. & Ellahi, B. (2016). *Evaluation Report Change Step: A Peer Mentoring Support Programme for Veterans in Wales and Listen In: A Support Programme for Families of Veterans in Wales. April 2016.* University of Chester.

Murrison, A. (2010). *Policy Paper. Fighting Fit: A mental health plan for servicemen and veterans.* London: HMSO.

National Institute for Clinical Excellence (NICE) (2005). *Post-traumatic stress disorder: The management of PTSD in adults and children in primary and secondary care.* London: NICE.

NHS England (2015). *Veterans: priority NHS treatment.* http://www.nhs.uk/NHSEngland/Militaryhealthcare/veterans-families-reservists/Pages/veterans.aspx (last accessed 30.8.2019).

Nottingham, R. & Bunn, S. (2016). *Postnote Number 518: Psychological Health of Military Personnel.* London: Parliamentary Office of Science and Technology.

Rowe, M., Murphy, D., Wessely, S. & Fear, N.T. (2013). Exploring the impact of deployment to Iraq on relationships. *Military Behavioral Health.* **1**, 13

Sayers, S.L., Farrow, V.A., Ross, J. & Oslin, D.W. (2009. Family problems among recently returned Military veterans referred for a mental health evaluation. *Journal of Clinical Psychiatry.* **70** (2), 163–70.

Soanes, C. & Stevenson, A. (2009). *Oxford Dictionary of English.* 2nd edn. Oxford: Oxford University Press.

Stevelink, S.A., Malcolm, E.M., Mason, C., Jenkins, S., Sundin, J. & Fear, N.T. (2014). The prevalence of mental health disorders in (ex-)military personnel with a physical impairment: a systematic review. *Occupational & Environmental Medicine.* http://doi.org/10.1136/oemed-2014-102207 (last accessed 30.8.2019).

van Hoorn, L.A., Jones, N., Busuttil, W., Fear, N.T., Wessely, S., Hunt, E. & Greenberg, N. (2013). Iraq and Afghanistan veteran presentations to Combat Stress, since 2003. *Occupational Medicine.* **63** (3), 238–41. http://doi.org/10.1093/occmed/kqt017 (last accessed 30.8.2019).

Whybrow, D., Jones, N. & Greenberg, N. (2015). Promoting organizational well-being: a comprehensive review of Trauma Risk Management. *Occupational Medicine.* http://doi.org/10.1093/occmed/kqv024 (last accessed 30.8.2019).

Chapter 10

Working with families affected by dementia

Mandy King

Introduction

Family carers provide the majority of support for people with dementia living at home and throughout the progression of the disease. Anyone who engages with someone who has dementia can, if they so wish, become part of their care. This helps keep memories fresh and true, and it ensures that the essence of the person with dementia is never lost. Family relationships are particularly important in enabling people living with dementia to experience wellbeing, maintain their identity and enhance their self-esteem. Alzheimer's Research UK (2015) define a carer as:

> ...anybody who looks after a family member, friend or neighbour who needs help because of illness, frailty or disability. All the care they give is unpaid, although they may be eligible for certain benefits. Anyone, of any age, can become a carer.

Across the world, there are an estimated 36 million people living with dementia and this figure is expected to almost double every 20 years, reaching 66 million by 2030 and 115 million by 2050 (WHO 2012). It is estimated that there are 850,000 people living with dementia in the UK, and 700,000 family and friends are caring for a person with dementia (Lewis *et al.* 2014).

Dementia is recognised within the UK as a significant health and social care issue that not only impacts on those living with dementia but also on their families, friends and carers. It is essential to find ways of working that will improve family carer support and offset the demands made by dementia care, which can jeopardise carers' own physical and mental wellbeing. The need to support carers of people with dementia is widely recognised within policy, which emphasises that people with dementia must be supported to continue engaging in everyday activities as long as they possibly can, and that they should be prevented from going into institutional settings prematurely (Welsh Government 2017, Department of Health 2012, 2015). Such a policy trend is in line with a person-centred approach, which is considered by many countries as good practice (WHO 2012).

As discussed later in this chapter, it is acknowledged across the UK that when families are given adequate information, support and care, it is possible for people with dementia to live well at home. UK legislation for carers has recently been updated, with the Care Act 2014 and Children and Families Act 2014 in England, the Carers (Scotland) Act 2016 and the Social Services & Well-being (Wales) Act 2014. All this legislation is intended to ensure that carers have carer assessments and services to meet their needs.

Throughout the chapter, the terms 'person/people with dementia (PWD)' and 'carer' are used. The word 'carer' denotes family members, friends and neighbours with caring responsibilities. This chapter explores what works to support carers of PWD, including providing information, support and psychosocial interventions.

Aims and learning outcomes

The aim of this chapter is to consider the needs of families or carers of people with dementia. Having completed this chapter, the reader will be able to:

- Assess the needs of carers or family members
- Consider an appropriate approach to take to help the family unit.

Being a carer for a person with dementia

Caring for a PWD can be both challenging and rewarding. It can change family relationships and impact on physical and psychological health (Alzheimer's Research UK 2015). The challenges faced by family carers are well documented and may include stress and social isolation (Barker & Board 2012, Ervin & Pallant 2015), financial difficulties, and physical and psychological problems (Lawrence *et al.* 2008). A carer is often thought of as the 'second invisible patient', as their needs are seen as secondary to those of the people they care for (Brodaty & Donkin 2009). The World Health Organization (2015) reports that carers of people living with dementia have a high mortality rate and are more likely to suffer from depression and anxiety disorders. Carers tend to experience a significant burden, with the difficulty of coping with the condition and behaviour changes of the person with dementia. However, the health and wellbeing of carers is critical to the quality of life for the PWD as well as helping to balance some of the deficits in the provision of health and social care. Zwaanswijk *et al.* (2013) argue that carers often have inadequate access to additional support and information and may therefore be poorly prepared to provide care. Yet, without the carer's support the PWD is likely to have a poorer quality of life and may need residential care sooner.

In the UK, government policy has highlighted the need to improve the lives of family carers, and current guidance recommends that family carers of people with dementia should have access to a range of psychosocial and practical support (NICE 2018). In June 2018, the National Institute for Health and Care Excellence (NICE) published a guideline, *Dementia: assessment, management and support for people living with dementia and their carers*. This guidance covers diagnosing and managing dementia (including Alzheimer's disease) and aims to improve care by making recommendations on training staff and helping carers to support people living with dementia. Key themes underpinning the guidelines include providing the carer with education, awareness and knowledge of dementia, and enhancing skills acquisition. All this requires the practitioner to share their skills and expertise in dementia care and ultimately help the carer understand and respond to changes in the behaviour of the PWD.

Nevertheless, the provision of support for carers is often fragmented and inadequate. Bunn *et al*. (2012) carried out a thematic analysis of over 100 qualitative studies of patient and carer experiences of dementia diagnosis and treatment and found that, although recent years had seen improvements in access to specialist diagnostic services, post-diagnosis support was still frequently considered inadequate by family carers. The Royal College of Nursing (RCN) project *Dignity in Dementia; Transforming General Hospital Care* (2011) highlighted the fact that involving family carers was highly instrumental in supporting improvements in care and was seen as a high priority by people with dementia, and carers and practitioners. Including and supporting carers of people with dementia will clearly lead to better outcomes for patients, carers and ultimately the professionals supporting them (Royal College of Nursing 2013).

Carer wellbeing is a key factor in hospital admissions, readmissions and delays in the transfer of care; and adequate carer support can lead to a reduction in the number of people with dementia requiring hospital admission (Conochie 2011).

Most commonly it is the spouse who takes on the role of family carer (Quinn *et al*. 2012) but when this is not possible the responsibility will fall to the adult child and this is mostly the daughter rather than the son (Ward-Griffin 2007). People take on the caring role for a number of reasons, including love, a sense of responsibility, expectation of family or social norms, cultural expectations or guilt (Murray 2014). Without this family care, many people with dementia would have a poorer quality of life and would be more likely to require a place in a nursing home or residential care home (Smits *et al*. 2007). It is important to recognise that the carer is the expert and has vast knowledge of the person with dementia (Department of Health 2015). The carer will see the person and not the dementia. When others become involved, they may have difficulty seeing who that person really is. Carers have an important role to play in helping the person with dementia keep their sense of identity and individuality especially when others become involved in their care. The carer is able to draw on their lived experiences of strategies to overcome the communication difficulties that are commonly experienced by the PWD.

Supporting carers of people with dementia

Person Centred Care (PCC) emerged in the 1990s as a framework in which to understand dementia and this has had a major influence on the way care is delivered across all dementia care settings. Kitwood (1997) introduced the concept of personhood into dementia care and proposed that we should value each individual as a unique person with individual rights and needs, arguing that the experience of dementia is unique to the individual and will depend on the interaction of many different factors. The environment can promote interactions that either maintain or destroy the personhood of the individual – and personhood is an important aspect of person-centred care: 'It is a standing or status that is bestowed on one human being, by others, in the context of relationship and social being. It implies recognition, respect and trust' (Kitwood 1997, p. 8).

A recent study (Chung *et al.* 2017) supports many of Kitwood's ideas and has provided empirical evidence that the personhood of those with dementia is maintained by family carers at home. Through a series of interviews, Chung *et al.*'s study concludes that carers face enormous challenges when the PWD loses interest in any activities that might keep either their mind or body active. Maintaining the PWD's previous identity, by encouraging activities and reaffirming their agency, can also benefit the carer's psychological wellbeing.

In the quote below, Christine Bryden is asking people around her to think about the whole person, not just the disease or deficits of the person with dementia. She explains what personhood means to her, as a person with dementia herself:

> How you relate to us has a big impact on the course of the disease. You can restore our personhood and give us a sense of being needed and valued. There is a Zulu saying that is very true, 'A person is a person through others'. Give us reassurance, hugs, support, a meaning in life. Value us for what we can still do and be, and make sure we retain social networks. It is very hard for us to be who we once were, so let us be who we are now – and realise the effort we are making to function. If you could see the damage inside our head, you would be amazed at the way we are managing despite missing bits in our brain.

(Taken from *Dancing with Dementia*, Bryden 2005, p. 107).

Christine Bryden is asking us to look past the medical diagnosis and see the person who remains, despite the dementia. To do this, we need to value the person she still is, and help her find ways to overcome the difficulties caused by the many symptoms of dementia. It is important to remember that each person with dementia will have different needs, based on who they are, their life history, personality, likes and dislikes, culture and beliefs, the severity of the dementia and their family history.

Christine Bryden suggests that enhancing or sustaining personhood relies upon relationships with others, the ways in which the person with dementia is able to remain connected and 'retain social networks'. Affection and a sense of still being loved (e.g. being given 'hugs') is important. Understandably, the carer may sometimes feel overwhelmed by the caring role and the routine tasks that are needed to ensure that the person with dementia is kept safe and physically well. The risk is that the carer may struggle to find time for meaningful interaction. Yet a sense of belonging, and feeling needed and valued by family members, is important – even when the person with dementia no longer recognises familiar faces or remembers the names of those closest to them. The contact with family members will still help the PWD to sustain the feeling that they belong, that they are still the mother, father or grandparent. The person with dementia can easily feel isolated and become lost. Families can help with this by providing a social network, keeping in touch and encouraging existing relationships to continue or by helping the person with dementia develop new relationships with members of the wider community. All this will help them hold on to their sense of identity, as the person that they are or once were.

To understand the lived experience of dementia, it is important to listen to the people with dementia themselves. Christine's story since her diagnosis shows us that there is hope. Since being diagnosed with dementia in 1995, she has been a strong advocate for people with dementia, addressing conferences around the world and appearing in the media.

In 2001 Christine Bryden was the first person with dementia to give a plenary address to the international conference of Alzheimer's Disease International (ADI). Then in 2003 she was the first person with dementia to be elected to the Board of Alzheimer's Disease International, a position she held for three years. She has given many talks and interviews in her home country of Australia, as well as elsewhere, such as Japan, New Zealand, Canada, UK, France, Israel, South Africa, Brazil, Dominican Republic, Taiwan, South Korea and Turkey. For more information about Christine and her remarkable story, visit her website: http://www.christinebryden.com/ (last accessed 31.8.2019).

Partnership working

This section will explore the potential of partnership working with people who have dementia and their carers, focusing on the importance of information, support and meaningful interventions. The need to think of carers as experts is highlighted in Government policy (Department of Health 2010, Marie Curie Cancer Care 2012). There are three key initiatives detailed below: the Triangle of Care; the relationship-centred care model and the use of Admiral Nurses in the UK. Principles from each of these approaches can be adapted and implemented in other practice arenas. Finally, there is an explanation of how carers can make use of the problem-solving model.

The Triangle of Care for dementia

The Triangle of Care for Dementia (Hannan *et al.* 2016) describes a therapeutic relationship between the person with dementia, the practitioner and the carer and aims to promote safety, support and communication and sustain wellbeing. The Triangle of Care for Dementia was originally developed in recognition of the need to improve carer involvement in acute hospital settings, but it is relevant and can be applied across all settings. The work was funded through the Royal College of Nursing Foundation and a collaborative effort between the Royal College of Nursing and the Carers Trust. It has been designed with input from carers, people with dementia and practitioners, with the support of Uniting Carers and Dementia UK. The Triangle of Care model of carer inclusion and support has proved to be very successful in mental health services, with over three-quarters of mental health providers in England involved in the project and the model being adapted for use in Scotland and Wales (Hannan *et al.* 2016).

The Triangle of Care for Dementia builds on the concept of relationship-centred care and emphasises 'the importance of relationships and interactions with others to the person with dementia, and their potential for promoting well-being in the delivery of person-centred care.' (NICE/SCIE 2006).

Table 10.1: The key standards to achieving a triangle of care *(Taken from RCN 2011)*

• Carers and the essential role they play are identified at first contact or as soon as possible thereafter.	• Carers' views and knowledge are sought, shared, used and regularly updated, as overall care plans and strategies to support treatment and care are developed
• Staff are 'carer aware' and trained in carer engagement strategies	• Staff welcome the valuable contribution carers can make and are mindful of carers' own needs as well as the needs of people with dementia
• Policy and practice protocols regarding confidentiality and sharing information, are in place	• Policies are in place that promote active carer involvement
• Defined post(s) responsible for carers are in place	• Carers leads or champions for all wards and teams who are skilled and knowledgeable about dementia
• A carer introduction to the service and staff is available, with a relevant range of information across the care pathway	• Carer information packs
• A range of carer support services is available	• Carer support systems • Evaluation processes

Relationship-centred care

My name is not dementia (Alzheimer's Society 2010) explored the definition of quality of life from the perspective of the person with dementia and the carer. Relationships were in the top three quality-of-life indicators for both groups. The relationship-centred care approach recognises the importance of the interpersonal and intrapersonal relationships that exist between the person with dementia and others around them. Nolan *et al.* (2008) argue that the senses framework can be used as a means of fostering supportive relationships in dementia care. The senses framework is underpinned by the belief that all those involved in caring (the older person, family carers, and paid or voluntary carers) should experience relationships that promote a sense of:

- Security – to feel safe within relationships; to receive good-quality care
- Belonging – to maintain present relationships and form new relationships; to feel a valued member of the community
- Continuity – to experience links and consistency
- Purpose – to have a personally valuable goal or goals
- Achievement – to make progress towards a desired goal or goals
- Significance – to feel that 'you' matter.

Admiral Nurses

Admiral Nurses were established as a result of the experiences of family carers. They are specialist dementia nurses who give expert practical, clinical and emotional support to families living with dementia. Admiral Nurses are named after Joseph Levy, who had vascular dementia and was known as 'Admiral Joe' because of his interest in sailing. An Admiral Nurse works across the different parts of the health and social care system, enabling the needs of family carers and people with dementia to be addressed in a coordinated way. There are approximately 200 Admiral Nurses working across the UK, supporting over 40,000 people affected by dementia to live more positively (Dementia UK 2018).

Bunn *et al.* (2016) undertook a systematic review of the literature relating to the scope and effectiveness of Admiral Nurses and a review of interventions. They concluded that community support for carers of people with dementia, such as that provided by Admiral Nurses, is valued by family carers, but the impact of such initiatives is not clearly established and requires more research. In addition to supporting families, Admiral Nurses work collaboratively with other health and social care professionals to educate and support them in raising the standard of care for people with dementia.

Helping carers to use a problem-solving approach

Carers need to feel involved, listened to and supported in their efforts to provide care. Carers ask for empathy and understanding (Cascioli *et al.* 2008). Behaviour changes can reduce quality of life for people with dementia as well as carers and can become a catalyst for the provision of more intensive support, including hospital and care home admission (Welsh Assembly Government 2010).

Healthcare professionals and carers can work together, using a problem-solving approach. The professional can work with the carer, explaining each step, and demonstrating professional understanding whilst also valuing the experiences of the carer as an expert. This partnership will facilitate the sharing of expertise and clinical skills and will also enable the carer to learn new strategies.

Table 10.2 provides an easily memorised guide to help avoid or overcome difficulties when using a problem-solving approach to care. You may find it helpful to use this 'PROBLEM' approach when supporting a carer in your own clinical practice. Work through each part with the carer and others involved. Then share your work, thoughts and ideas with colleagues.

Table 10.2: A problem-solving approach.

P	PINPOINT what the problem really is. Ask yourself who is this a problem for and why is this a problem? Consider your reaction to the problem. When does the problem happen? Is there a particular trigger, like time of day, or when dressing or washing? Break the problem down into small bite-size pieces. It will be easier to tackle than one big complex problem.
R	Be RESOURCEFUL. Think of as many ways of solving this problem as you can. What has already been tried? Why didn't it work? Make a list, use your imagination and write down everything that comes into your mind.
O	Consider all the different OPTIONS that are available to you. Go through your list and make a note of the pros and cons. What are the advantages and disadvantages of trying to change the behaviour?
B	BE patient. Sometimes you might decide to try one thing and it does not work, so you will want to try another. Sometimes you may try more than one course of action at a time.
L	LISTEN to and LOOK at the person with dementia, at both their verbal and non-verbal communication. What might be the underlying cause for the behaviour? Listening to experiences will help you decide which action to take first. You may find it useful to share and discuss the problem in a carers' support group or with family members.
E	ENLIST the help of others. As soon as you have decided upon a course of action, you can draw up a detailed plan of what to do and consider who might be able to help.
M	MAKE your plan work. Make it happen, and remember that every problem you experience is a learning opportunity and it will help you overcome future difficulties.

Providing information and support

The Carers Trust commissioned a study in 2012 that aimed to 'understand more about the caring journey undertaken by carers of people with dementia and the challenges they face' (Newbronner *et al.* 2013). One of the main findings was that there was a lack of information and support for carers throughout the whole journey. There are a number of ways of offering information and support, including the use of memory cafés, reminiscence and life story work and cognitive stimulation therapy for carers.

Illustrative case study

> Mr and Mrs Thomas are retired teachers and have been married for 45 years. They have one daughter who lives overseas.
>
> When Mrs Thomas went with her husband, Paul, to the memory clinic she was told that he had a type of dementia and that this was probably due to Alzheimer's disease. The doctor explained that it was a kind of brain damage, which would continue to get worse. She was told it was incurable but medication would be available if Mr Thomas became 'too difficult to cope with'.
>
> The doctor gave Mrs Thomas some leaflets about research into Alzheimer's disease. He said it might be possible for Mr Thomas to take part in a trial for a new drug that was being tested.

A diagnosis of dementia should be delivered in a compassionate and thoughtful manner, using a person-centred approach (Lee & Weston 2011). You may have concluded that Mr and Mrs Thomas will feel a sense of relief now that they have a name for Mr Thomas's condition. The period before diagnosis can be uncertain and a time of anxiety, knowing that there is something wrong but unsure what. Mr and Mrs Thomas now have a medical name for what is wrong, and they can begin to think about the future.

Helping people come to terms with their diagnosis and understand the disease process, and make decisions and plan ahead, is critical in supporting them to live well with dementia (Aminzadeh *et al.* 2007). As yet, there is no known cure for dementia. It is therefore understandable that, following a diagnosis of dementia, there is an acceptance that not much can be done to alleviate the disease. However, an early diagnosis will enable Mr and Mrs Thomas to work with the healthcare practitioner to plan and set goals for future care and make decisions about post-diagnostic support (Della Penna *et al.* 2002).

In the illustrative case study, the doctor provides some information on research into Alzheimer's disease. It is considered best practice to provide written information covering signs, symptoms, the course and prognosis of dementia, possible treatments, available services and signposting towards legal and financial advice (NICE/SCIE 2006). Studies show that people affected by dementia find it difficult to access information about their diagnosis, are unsure who to ask for support and what services are available

(Fontaine *et al.* 2011). Whilst there is no cure for dementia, there are medications available that can benefit the majority of people in the early to moderate stages of dementia. These treatments can improve the quality of life by enhancing cognitive functioning and increasing the person's ability to cope with everyday life. The doctor in the case study mentions that medications are available for times when Mr Thomas becomes difficult. Thus, there is an expectation that Mr Thomas will indeed become difficult and will need medication to control his behaviour in the future.

Mrs Thomas will need help to understand the changes in his emotional ability and cognitive functions and the way in which changes in his behaviour are linked to dementia. Helping the carer to understand the lived experience of dementia (in other words, what it might be like to live with dementia) will help them to accept and understand that the person with dementia can't help what is happening.

Carers will experience a wide range of emotions (possibly including guilt, grief, anxiety and depression) and they will need support to understand their own emotions and to cope with them. Carers also need support to learn to provide personal and intimate care for the PWD. This is often something they have never had to do for another adult. Carers need to be able to feel confident in caring and need the right education and skills to help them care well. Mental health practitioners can:

- Enhance the carer's own knowledge and skills, rather than telling them what to do
- Help carers who need to navigate health and social care systems, as this is often unfamiliar ground
- Offer carers support to look after their own emotional and physical health needs and to take some time out for themselves.

Parkinson *et al.* (2017) suggest that a coherent approach to 'resilience building' is vital in order to meet the needs of the carer. This involves reviewing current databases to gain a deeper understanding of what works when supporting family members and carers of people with dementia. For healthcare professionals who wish to provide biopsychosocial and service support that will augment carer resilience and support carers of people with dementia, five key themes emerge: extending social assets, strengthening key psychological resources, maintaining physical health status, safeguarding quality of life and having key resources available in a timely manner.

Dementia-Friendly Cafés (also known as Memory Cafés)

Facilitating activities that are enjoyed by both PWDs and carers is another intervention strategy that can help reduce carer burden (Searson *et al.* 2008).

Dementia-Friendly Cafés were originally set up to provide a social opportunity for people with dementia. At these meeting places, they could find information and support, meet other people and improve their general wellbeing. Cafés provide stimulating activities for carers and people with dementia, which can help prevent boredom and aid relaxation. These activities may include, for example, live music, sing-alongs, quizzes, painting, memory box work, massage and reflexology.

1. Memory cafés are usually held on a regular basis, either once a week, once a fortnight, or once a month. Most are located in places that are easy to access, such as community centres, village halls or local hotels.
2. Tables are laid out 'café style' and refreshments are served.
3. Memory cafés are run by people (including volunteers) who have experience and training in dementia. A healthcare professional is often available to provide one-to-one advice and support.

Dementia-Friendly Leeds, in collaboration with Leeds Trinity University, gathered feedback from dementia-friendly groups and cafés across Leeds. This report set out to identify the successes and knowledge of the dementia-friendly groups consulted and to share their insights across all dementia-friendly groups in Leeds (Dementia Action Alliance 2007). The report findings included:

- As well as people with dementia, carers very much look forward to the groups.
- The groups provided an opportunity to socialise with other carers, improve wellbeing and 'just get out of the house'.
- Another benefit was awareness being raised in the wider community. The report provides several examples of this, including the following: 'a police community support officer regularly supporting a man living with dementia. He often walked around the village and became disorientated. Now the officer assists him to attend the group' (Dementia Action Alliance 2017).
- Other benefits included peer support from other carers, information provision and support from the volunteer café coordinators.

Reminiscence and life story work

Reminiscence aims to improve communication with older people by engaging them in conversation using sensory stimuli as triggers to spark memories. People with dementia can engage and communicate very successfully if the conversation sparks a memory from their past and they are given the opportunity to recall the details of that memory. For people with short-term memory loss, conversing about the present can be very stressful. In contrast, reminiscence enables the PWD to remember and converse about the past, sharing their memories of life and maintaining their identity beyond the dementia. A study by Woods *et al.* (2012) assessed the effectiveness and cost-effectiveness of joint reminiscence groups for people with dementia and their family caregivers, compared with usual care. However, the findings did not support the effectiveness or cost-effectiveness of joint reminiscence groups for people with dementia and their carers, as there were benefits for the PWD but the carers found this experience upsetting.

Family involvement in life story work is one way in which care delivery and communication can be personalised and enhanced (Keady & Swarbrick 2011). Life story work is a psychotherapeutic intervention that involves working with a person with dementia, family members and friends to record key moments of their past and present lives, usually in a scrapbook, photo album or video album. The book or album will play an important role in providing person-centred care and support.

It is often possible to find out something simple from the person's past, such as where they lived or what they did for a living. Using this as a starting point, you can then reminisce with them, using pictures and objects relating to this part of their life. As the process continues, more and more memories will be recovered and new ones will emerge. This helps family, friends and care workers to build up a unique picture of the person – and helps them to communicate with you. As the dementia progresses, life story work can play an increasingly important role in helping to stimulate conversation, especially when meeting the person for the first time.

The Life Story Network (LSN) works with a range of partner organisations and individuals, promoting the value of using life stories to 'improve the quality of life and wellbeing of people and communities, particularly those marginalised or made vulnerable through ill health or disability' (http://www.lifestorynetwork.org.uk/).

Cognitive stimulation therapy

Cognitive stimulation therapy (CST) is a well-established group psychosocial intervention for people with dementia. It is a brief treatment programme for people with mild to moderate dementia and it involves 14 or more sessions of themed activities, which typically run twice weekly. Sessions aim to actively stimulate and engage people with dementia, whilst providing a learning environment and the social benefits of being part of a group. The effects of CST appear to be comparable to those reported with the currently available anti-dementia drugs. UK Government NICE guidance (NICE 2006) on the management of dementia recommends the use of group CST for people with mild to moderate dementia, irrespective of drug treatments received. Further information on CST can be found at http://www.cstdementia.com/.

More recently, a one-to-one individualised version of CST, known as iCST, has been developed. Sessions follow similar themes and principles to group CST and this form of therapy can be offered by family carers or health professionals. The individualised version, iCST, is considered a useful tool when encouraging people with dementia and their carers to communicate (Leung *et al.* 2017). There is evidence that iCST delivered by the family carer can benefit both the person with dementia and their carer.

SONAS: Activating the Potential to Communicate (APC)

It is well known that PWD can spend many hours with only minimal interaction with others. This is often a result of communication difficulties experienced both by the person with dementia and the carer, possibly resulting in the PWD becoming isolated, withdrawn and lost. The person with dementia may have difficulty in expressing (both verbally and non-verbally) who they once were, who they are today and who they wish to be in the future. To provide good-quality dementia care, it is essential to see the person beyond the dementia and deliver care that is empathic and respectful. To do this, we need to find a way to activate each individual's potential to communicate; to help the person be who they truly are, to express their likes, their dislikes and their personality, and help them to use the abilities and potential they have retained.

Practitioners can work with carers to raise awareness of sensory stimulation as a possible intervention to improve the PWD's quality of life. Sonas APC (now known as Engaging dementia, https://engagingdementia.ie/) values the individuality and inherent dignity of older people and believes that the human need for love, friendship and relationship is met through communication. This approach has been shown to enhance the lives of older people with impaired communication, especially those with moderate to severe dementia (Strøma *et al.* 2018). It strives to help older people with unmet communication needs to realise their communicative potential and experience an enhanced quality of life.

The Sonas approach is grounded in the right of each older person to respect, choice and privacy. A Sonas session involves stimulating all five senses (hearing, sight, touch, taste and smell). Different sensory stimulation interventions are used for the PWD, to increase alertness, reduce agitation and improve quality of life. When carers understand the nature of communication, and how it is affected by conditions such as dementia, this gives them a greater insight into how to connect with the person they care for. The Sonas approach can therefore potentially offer a great improvement in quality of life and environment for both the carer and the PWD.

Reflection

- When you next work with a person with dementia, or memory problems, how might you involve the family or carers in your discussions?
- What approach do you think would be helpful?

Conclusion

Family and friends play a vital role in the life of a person living with dementia, helping the PWD maintain their personhood and enabling them to continue to live a full and meaningful life within their community. Becoming a carer involves taking on new roles, tasks and responsibilities and may involve a change in the relationship with the person with dementia. Support for carers is therefore vital. Family work includes creating opportunities for interventions that can support relationship-centred models such as reminiscence, life story work and cognitive stimulation therapy.

References

Alzheimer's Research UK (2015). *Women and Dementia: A Marginalised Majority*. Cambridge: Alzheimer's Research UK.

Alzheimer's Society (2010). *My name is not dementia: People with dementia discuss quality of life indicator*. London: Alzheimer's Society.

Aminzadeh, F., Byszewski, A., Molnar, F.J. & Eisner, M. (2007). Emotional impact of dementia diagnosis: exploring persons with dementia and caregivers' perspectives. *Aging & Mental Health*. **11** (3), 281–90.

Barker, S. & Board, M. (2012). *Dementia Care in Nursing. Transforming Nursing Practice Series*. London: RCN Publishing.

Brodaty, H. & Donkin, M. (2009). Family caregivers of people with dementia. *Dialogues Clinical Neuroscience*. **11** (2), 217–28

Bryden, C. (2005). *Dancing with Dementia*. London: Jessica Kingsley Publishers.

Bunn. F., Goodman, C., Sworn, K., Rait, G., Brayne, C., Robinson, L., McNeilly, E. & Iliffe, S. (2012). Psychosocial factors that shape patient and carer experiences of dementia diagnosis and treatment: a systematic review of qualitative studies. *PLoS Medicine*. https://www.ncbi.nlm.nih.gov/pubmed/23118618 (last accessed 31.8.2019).

Bunn. F., Goodman, C., Sworn, K., Rait, G., Brayne, C., Robinson, L., McNeilly, E. & Iliffe, S. (2016) Specialist nursing and community support for the carers of people with dementia living at home: an evidence synthesis. *Health and Social Care in the Community*. **24** (1), 48–67.

Cascioli, T.R., Al-Madfai, H., Oborne, P. & Phelps, S. (2008). An evaluation of the needs and service usage of family carers of people with dementia. *Quality in Ageing – Policy, practice and research*. **9**(2), 18–27.

Chung, P.Y.F., Ellis-Hill, C. & Coleman, P. (2017). Supporting activity engagement by family carers at home: maintenance of agency and personhood in dementia. *International Journal of Qualitative Studies on Health and Well-being*. **12** (1). doi: 10.1080/17482631.2016.1267316

Conochie, G. (2011). *Supporting Carers: The Case for Change*. (The Princess Royal Trust for Carers and Crossroads Care). http://static.carers.org/files/supporting-carers-the-case-for-change-5728.pdf (last accessed 25.9.2019).

Della Penna, R.D., Heumann, K.S., Gade, G. & Venohr, I. (2002). Evidence-based clinical vignettes from the Care Management Institute: Alzheimer's disease and dementia. *The Permanente Journal*. **6** (2), 43–50.

Dementia Action Alliance (2007). *Dementia Cafés and Groups in Leeds Report 2017: Sharing challenges, successes, resources and best practice across groups for people with dementia in Leeds.*

Dementia UK (2018). *Working Together to Face Dementia*. http://www.dementiauk.org/wp-content/uploads/2018/01/DementiaUK_A4_20pp_2017-AnnualReview_WEB.compressed.pdf (last accessed 31.8.2019).

Department of Health (DH) (2010). *Recognised, valued and supported: Next steps for the carers strategy*. London: DH.

Department of Health (DH) (2012). *Prime Minister's challenge on dementia: Delivering major Improvements in dementia care and research by 2015*. London: DH.

Department of Health (DH) (2015). *Prime Minister's challenge on dementia 2020*. London: DH.

Ervin, K., J. & Pallant, J. (2015). A rural study of carer well-being. *Australasian Journal on Ageing*. **34** (4), 235–40

Fontaine, J.L., Brooker, D., Bray, J. & Milosevic, S.K. (2011). *A local evaluation of dementia advisers (National Demonstrator Site): Worcestershire report for Dementia Adviser Service implementation team*. Worcester: University of Worcester.

Hannan, R., Thompson, R., Worthington, A. & Rooney, P. (2016). *The Triangle of Care Carers Included: A Guide to Best Practice for Dementia Care*. London: Carers Trust

Keady, J. & Swarbrick, C. (2011). Dementia care: family and significant others. *Nursing and Residential Care.* **13** (11) 546–47.

Kitwood, T. (1997). *Dementia Reconsidered: The person comes first*. Buckingham: Open University Press.

Lawrence, V., Murray, J., Samsi, K. & Banerjee, S. (2008). Attitudes and support needs of Black Caribbean, South Asian and White British carers of people with dementia in the UK. *The British Journal of Psychiatry.* **193** (3), 240–46.

Lee, L. & Weston, W.W. (2011), Disclosing a diagnosis of dementia: Helping learners to break bad news. *Canadian Family Physician.* **57** (7), 851–52.

Leung, P., Yates, L., Orgeta, V., Hamidi, F. & Orrell, M. (2017). The experiences of people with dementia and their carers participating in individual cognitive stimulation therapy. *International Journal of Geriatric Society.* **32** (12).

Lewis, F., Karlsberg Schaffer, S., Sussex, J., O'Neill, P. & Cockcroft, L. (2014). *Trajectory of Dementia in the UK – Making a Difference.* Report produced the Office of Health Economics for Alzheimer's Research UK.

Marie Curie Cancer Care (2012). *Committed to carers: Supporting carers of people at end of life report.* London: Marie Curie Cancer Care.

Murray A. (2014). The effect of dementia on patients, informal carers and nurses. *Nursing Older People.* **26** (5), 27–31. doi: 10.7748/nop.26.5.27.e573.

National Institute for Health and Clinical Excellence (NICE) and Social Care Institute for Excellence (SCIE) (2006). *Dementia: Supporting people with dementia and their carers in health and social care. CG42*. London: NICE/SCIE.

National Institute for Health and Clinical Excellence (NICE) (2018). *Dementia: assessment, management and support for people living with dementia and their carers. NICE guideline* [NG97]. London.

Newbronner, L., Chamberlain, R., Borthwick, R. *et al.* (2013). *A road less rocky: supporting carers of people with dementia*. Research Report. Carers Trust.

Nolan, M., Davies, S., Ryan, T. & Keady, J. (2008). Relationship-centred care and the 'Senses' framework. *Journal of Dementia Care.* **16**, 26–28.

Parkinson, M., Carr, S.M., Rushmer, R. & Abley, C. (2017). Investigating what works to support family carers of people with dementia: a rapid realist review. *Journal of Public Health.* **39** (4), e290–e301, https://doi.org/10.1093/pubmed/fdw100 (last accessed 30.9.2019).

Quinn, C., Clare, L., McGuinness, T. & Woods, R.T. (2012). The impact of relationships, motivations, and meanings on dementia caregiving outcomes. *International Psychogeriatrics.* **24**, 1816–26. doi:10.1017/S1041610212000889

Royal College of Nursing (RCN) (2011). *Project Dignity in Dementia; Transforming General Hospital Care*. London: RCN Publishing.

Royal College of Nursing (RCN) (2013). *Dementia: Commitment to the Care of People with Dementia in Hospital Settings*. London: RCN Publishing.

Searson, R., Hendry, A.M., Ramachandran, R., Burns, A. & Purandare N. (2008). Activities enjoyed by patients with dementia together with their spouses and psychological morbidity in carers. *Aging & Mental Health.* **12** (2), 276–82. doi: 10.1080/13607860801956977.

Smits, C.H., de Lange, J., Dröes, R.M., Meiland, F., Vernooij-Dassen, M. & Pot, A.M. (2007). Effects of combined intervention programmes for people with dementia living at home and their caregivers: a systematic review. *International Journal of Geriatric Psychiatry.* **22** (12), 1181–93. doi:10.1002/gps.1805.

Strøma, B.S., Benth, J.S. & Engedalc, K. (2018). Impact of the Sonas Programme on Communication over a Period of 24 Weeks in People with Moderate-to-Severe Dementia. *Dementia & Geriatric Cognitive Disorders Extra.* **8**, 238–47.

Ward-Griffin, C. (2007). Mother-adult daughter relationships within dementia care: a critical analysis. *Journal of Family Nursing.* **13** (1), 13–32.

Welsh Assembly Government (2012). *1000 Lives: Improving Dementia Care.* The Heath Foundation. http://www.1000livesplus.wales.nhs.uk/sitesplus/documents/1011/How%20to%20%2815%29%20 Dementia%20%28Feb%202011%29%20Web.pdf (last accessed 30.9.2019).

Welsh Government (2017). *The Dementia Action Plan for Wales.* Cardiff: Welsh Government.

Woods, R.T., Bruce, E., Edwards, R.T., Elvish, R., Hoare, Z., Hounsome, B., Keady, J., Moniz-Cook, E.D., Orgeta, V., Orrell, M., Rees, J. & Russell, I.T. (2012). REMCARE: reminiscence groups for people with dementia and their family caregivers – effectiveness and cost-effectiveness pragmatic multicentre randomised trial. *Health Technology Assessment.* **16** (48), v–xv, 1–116. doi: 10.3310/hta16480.

World Health Organization (WHO) (2012). *Dementia: A public health priority.* Switzerland: World Health Organization and Alzheimer's Disease International, World Health Organization Press.

Zwaanswijk, M., Peeters, J.M., Beek, A.P., Meerveld, J.H. & Francke, A.L. (2013). Informal caregivers of people with dementia: problems, needs and support in the initial stage and in subsequent stages of dementia: a questionnaire survey. *The Open Nursing Journal.* **7**, 6–13.

Index

Admiral Nurses 133
adult mental health services, family-centred care in 9–11
alcohol guidelines 103
alcohol misuse 103–112
assessment tools 24–27, 73
attachment 71
attachment domain 54

bioecological model of human development 5
bipolar affective disorder 47
Bowlby, John 2, 71

Care Programme Approach (CPA) 85
carer burden 20, 21
carer burden, effects of 22
carer, definition of 127
carers, well-being of 22, 129
caring for a person with dementia 128
caring, positive impact of 23
case management 94
child-focused interventions 42
children and young people's mental health services (CAMHS), family-centred care in 6–9, 40
children of parents with mental health issues (COPMI), needs of 41
Cognitive Behavioural Conjoint Therapy 119, 120
cognitive stimulation therapy (CST) 138
communication 110, 111
communication difficulties in dementia 139
community intensive therapy team (CITT) 9
community services 45
confidentiality 35
cultural diversity 23

dementia 10
dementia, families affected by 127–140
dementia-friendly cafés 136
dementia nurses 133
dementia, supporting carers of people with 130, 136
discipline/expectation domain 55
domain clarity 60
domains framework in the context of CAMHS inpatient nursing 63, 64
drug misuse 103

emotional resilience 46
experience of caring 20
exploratory domain 56, 59
expressed emotion 17, 18, 19, 23

families and carers, needs of 15–28
families, types of viii
family carers' experiences in a secure context 86
family interactional processes 51–65
family intervention in psychosis 32, 33
family interventions in perinatal context 77, 78
family interventions in substance misuse 108, 109, 111
family, meaning of viii
Family Questionnaire (FQ) 26
family structure 70
Family Talk Intervention 42

family work, benefits of vii
family-centred care (FCC) in children's services 1–9
family-centred care, benefits of 3
family-centred care, challenges to 4
family-centred care, context of 2
family-centred care, elements of 3
family-centred care, philosophy of 2
family-focused interventions for parents with mental health issues 45
feeding pattern of the baby 76
forensic settings, support and services for carers in 89

healthcare delivery, change in 16

information sharing 34, 35
inpatient services 45

KGV symptom scale 25, 26
Knowledge About Schizophrenia Interview (KASI) 27

life story work 137, 138

maternal death by suicide 68
maternal mental health problems 67
maternal perinatal mental health 69
memory cafés 136
mental health nursing, family-centred care in 1–11
mental health problems, causes of 17
mental health problems, long-term impact of 16
military deployment, impact on families 118
military personnel and veterans, mental health service provision for 116, 117, 118
military veterans, working with 115–124
miscarriage 77

Neonatal Behavioural Assessment Scale (NBAS) 76
nurse–family partnerships 6

open dialogue approach 94, 95

parental mental health problems, impact on child 70
parent–child interaction, observation of 75
parent-focused interventions 43
parents with mental health issues 39–48
parents with mental health issues, experiences of 42
partnership working with people who have dementia and their carers 131
paternal depression 70
paternal perinatal mental health 69
perinatal assessment 72
perinatal mental health 67–79
perinatal mental health interventions 74
Person Centred Care (PCC) 130
personhood 130
Platt report 2
postnatal depression 68
post-traumatic stress disorder 75, 117, 118, 120
practitioner skills 46
problem-solving 35, 36, 37
problem-solving approach 134
professional skills in substance misuse 110

psycho-education 33, 34, 35, 47, 92
psychosis 19, 31–38
psychosocial family interventions 9
psychosocial interventions 91

recovery approach 74
relationship between the professional and the person and family 110
relationship-centred care 133
Relative Assessment Interview (RAI) 25
reminiscence 137
risk assessment 94

safety domain 54
schizophrenia 21
secure care, impact on families and children 90
secure mental health services, family support and involvement in 83–96
self-harm 61
self-management and recovery training 107
sensory stimulation interventions 139
separation anxiety 2
sleep deprivation 76
Social Domains Framework 52–65
Social Functioning Scale (SFS) 26
stillbirth 77
substance misuse 103–112
substance misuse, effects of 106
substance misuse, effects on family 107
substance misuse interventions 107, 108
substance misuse, reasons for 105, 106
substance misuse stigma 104, 105
substance misuse terminology 104, 105
support groups for children of parents with mental health issues 43
support groups for parents with mental health issues 43

therapeutic alliance 10, 65
transtheoretical model of change 111
Triangle of Care 85
Triangle of Care for Dementia 132

veteran, definition of 115
veterans' mental health 118